TRUSTED HOME
REMEDIES

More Than 1,000 Simple Treatments
for EVERYDAY HEALTH PROBLEMS

Reader's
Digest

New York/Montreal

Previously published as *1,801 Home Remedies*

ISBN 978-1-62145-546-2

The Library of Congress has catalogued the original edition of this book as
follows:
1,801 Home Remedies: trustworthy treatments for everyday health
problems / Readers Digest.-- 1st ed.
    p. cm.
  ISBN 978-1-62145-546-2 (paperback)
  ISBN 978-1-62145-547-9 (ePub)
  1. Therapeutics--Popular works. 2. Self-care, Health. I. Title: One
thousand eight hundred and one home remedies. II. Reader's Digest
Association.
  RM122.5.A15 2003
  616.02'4--dc22
                        2003020949

Address any comments about *Home Remedies* to:
Reader's Digest Adult Trade Publishing
44 South Broadway
White Plains, NY 10601

Visit our website at rd.com

Printed in Singapore

Note to Readers
The information in this book should not be substituted for, or used to alter,
any medical treatment or therapy without your doctor's advice.

10 9 8 7 6 5 4 3 2 1

Contributors

Bookside Press

    Editors Edward B. Claflin, E. A. Tremblay
    Writers Matthew Hoffman, Eric Metcalf
    Researchers Janel Bogert, Elizabeth Shimer

Project Editor Marianne Wait
Copy Editor Jeanette Gingold
Indexer Ellen Brennan
Illustrators Harry Bates, Inkgraved Illustration;
    Cindy Jeftovic
Designer Richard Kershner

Medical Advisors

Carolyn Dean, M.D., N.D. Consultant, Integrative Medicine,
    City Island, New York

Mitchell A. Fleisher, M.D. Clinical Instructor, University of Virginia
    Health Sciences Center and the Medical College of Virginia;
    Family Physician, Private Practice, Nellysford, Virginia

Larrian Gillespie, M.D. Retired Assistant Clinical Professor
    of Urology and Urogynecology, Beverly Hills, California

Chris Kammer, D.D.S. Center for Cosmetic Dentistry,
    Madison, Wisconsin

Chris Meletis, N.D. Chief Medical Officer and Director
    of Education Affairs, Pearl Clinic Professor of Natural
    Pharmacology, National College of Naturopathic Medicine,
    Portland, Oregon

Lylas G. Mogk, M.D. Henry Ford Visual Rehabilitation
    & Research Center, Grosse Pointe and Livonia, Michigan

Zorba Paster, M.D. Professor of Family Medicine, Dean Medical
    Center, University of Wisconsin–Madison

Ricki Pollycove, M.D., M.H.S. Clinical Faculty, University of
    California School of Medicine; Private Practice of Gynecology,
    San Francisco, California

David B. Posner, M.D. Chief of Gastroenterology,
Mercy Medical Center, Baltimore, Maryland; Assistant Professor
    of Medicine, University of Maryland School of Medicine

Adrienne Rencic, M.D., Ph.D. Attending Dermatologist, Mercy
    Medical Center, Baltimore, Maryland; Clinical Instructor,
    University of Maryland Medical System

Kevin R. Stone, M.D. Orthopedic Surgeon and Founder and
    Chairman of The Stone Foundation for Sports Medicine and
    Arthritis Research and the Stone Clinic, San Francisco, California

Cathryn Tobin, M.D. Pediatrician, Private Practice, Markham,
    Ontario

Trusted Home Remedies

Table of

Contents

Using Home Remedies

At the age of 85, Adelia Liercke of Clarence, Iowa, still takes the same cough medicine that her mother and father used—a mixture of honey, onion, and lemon juice. When Betty W. Bishop of Hampton, Florida, gets a boil, she spreads the membrane of a boiled egg across it to "draw out the core"—a trick that her mom taught her. When Cindy Leaf of Glenfield, New York, detects the beginning of a cold, she mixes up a potent medicine brew using a family recipe for "nature's penicillin" that includes 24 fresh cloves of garlic.

Nearly every family has some home remedies that have been passed along from one generation to the next. Their origins are lost in the mists of time. Who was the first grandmother to serve peppermint tea to a sick grandchild? Why did a woodsman decide to crush the leaves of a jewelweed plant and spread it on poison ivy? Who was the first cook to discover that chicken soup can help you recover from the common cold?

Considering how often favorite home remedies have been used to cure everyday ailments and relieve pain, it's a pity we don't know the names of the originators. They deserve Nobel Prizes in Practical Medicine. But maybe there's a better way to honor their contributions. We can *use* the home remedies that they so generously passed along to us.

More Than One Thousand Remedies—Right Here!

Home remedies begin at home—and often that's where the secrets remain.

But with this book, you're opening the doors to thousands of homes, discovering the cornucopia of remedies that have been passed along for hundreds of years.

Some of the remedies came to us by mail from local readers. But that was only the beginning. We also uncovered folk cures used by early American pioneers, acupressure treatments of Chinese doctors, and the healing methods of tribal shamans.

We discovered the leading home remedies endorsed by naturopathic doctors and massage therapists, herbalists and homeopathic physicians, specialists in cardiovascular medicine and favorite family doctors. Our search for these remedies carried us through history, from the era of Hippocrates to the battlefields of World War I and the backyard gardens of twenty-first century herbal healers.

Selecting the Best

Though we cast a wide net, our final selection of the best home remedies was a selective process. To be honest, a number of traditional home remedies didn't make the cut because they were just too . . . well . . . strange. The asafetida bag, once a cherished cure for colds, has a smell so noxious that it's remembered with horror by those who used it. Other old remedies are so odd and complex that they aren't worth passing on, except for curiosity's sake. An Appalachian cure for warts, for instance, was to rub a potato on the wart, place the potato in a sack, and leave the sack at a fork in the road.

Of course, any remedy that does no harm might also do some good, especially when administered by someone who has a gentle, healing touch and cares deeply for the patient. But when we cast out the oddest, least-credible, most-complicated, and slightly risky, we were left with the wonderful (and sometimes wondrous) remedies that you'll find in this book. Each of these remedies was then carefully reviewed by our board of advisors—including physicians, highly qualified specialists, and naturopathic doctors—to ensure that they are safe for you to use as recommended.

Every remedy in this book was carefully reviewed by our board of advisors to ensure that they are safe for you to use as recommended.

All Within Reach

As you read about the home remedies in this book—and start to use them yourself—you'll probably begin to recall tried-and-true healing techniques that come from your own family. But we've all gotten so used to blood tests, X rays, high-potency (and high-cost) prescription drugs, and all the other trappings of modern medicine that we tend to forget, or neglect, our amazing legacy of at-home cures. Time-tested remedies are just as useful today as they ever were. The tricks you learned from your parents and grandparents, like sprinkling meat tenderizer on a bee sting or putting a soothing tea bag on tired eyes, aren't replacements for high-tech treatments, of course. But you can count on them to feel better fast—and, in many cases, to prevent small problems from turning into bigger ones.

There's something almost magical about watching a burn heal when you follow your grandmother's advice and apply a dab of aloe vera gel.

There's something very satisfying about watching a burn heal almost like magic when you follow your grandmother's advice and apply a dab of aloe vera gel. Or when you inhale the scent of lavender and feel anxiety slip away. But nostalgia isn't the reason doctors continue to recommend home treatments. They recommend them because they work.

All those drugs in your medicine cabinet? At least 25 percent of them contain active ingredients that are similar or identical to those found in plants. The active substance in aspirin—one of the world's most popular medications—was originally derived from white willow bark. The decongestant ephedrine is based on chemicals in the ephedra plant. The heart drug digitalis is derived from the foxglove. The cancer drug taxol comes from the Pacific yew tree. In fact, big drug makers continually send teams of scientists to remote locations to scour the countryside for medically promising chemicals.

Finding What Works

In current medical practice, traditional healing techniques are sometimes neglected, but with luck they're never forgotten. Physical therapists use the same hot and cold treatments that were popular among Native American tribes—treatments that often work better than aspirin, with none of the side effects. Kitchen cuts certainly heal better when you apply a dab of triple antibiotic. But guess what? A slathering of honey does the same thing and may help the cut heal faster.

Molly Hopkins, a 60-year-old landscape designer in Albuquerque, New Mexico, discovered firsthand that traditional treatments are sometimes superior to their conventional counterparts. "I used to get sinus infections every time I got a cold, and then I had to take antibiotics," she says. Her friend, a family physician, told her to start taking echinacea at the first sign of sniffles. "I haven't had a serious cold since—and no sinus infections at all," she says.

Most of us use traditional cures for minor aches and pains, but doctors at top research institutions now realize that they also work for some of our most serious health threats. Take diabetes. Millions of Americans need injections or oral drugs to keep blood sugar levels stable. Those who also eat a clove of garlic daily may naturally lower blood sugar and with it their doses of medicine. Depression is another condition that frequently requires medication, yet studies show that the herb St. John's wort may be just as effective as drugs for mild to moderate cases. And because the active ingredient (hypericin) enters the body gradually, it almost never causes the side effects common with prescription drugs, such as sexual dysfunction or low energy.

Many of the most popular at-home cures, such as yogurt for yeast infections or chamomile tea for insomnia, have been used for generations. Others—what you might call "future traditions" that will hopefully be passed along to your children and grandchildren—are being developed all the time.

- Researchers at Cincinnati Children's Hospital Medical Center recently found that duct tape, that all-purpose household fix-it, causes warts to disappear in just a few days.

- Creams laced with the herb arnica help bruises heal faster and with less pain because they contain natural painkilling and anti-inflammatory compounds.

- Zinc improves skin blemishes in about a third of people who take it—and this mighty mineral is just as effective as the drug tetracycline at healing severe acne.

"Why should I wait three weeks to see a doctor and pay a fortune for a prescription when I know there are some problems I can treat myself?" asks Margie Baker, a therapist in Tucson, Arizona. "You don't have to be a rocket scientist to know that a baking-soda bath is good for sunburn. I grew up in Florida, for goodness' sakes. I know it works."

The Commonsense Approach

While the remedies in this book comprise a veritable treasure trove of health solutions, there's nothing like good judgment when it comes to using any home remedy. Sometimes you need to be on the lookout for signs of more serious problems.

Clara Boxer made the kind of mistake doctors always worry about. A 53-year-old Philadelphia accountant, she'd been suffering from occasional dizziness, usually in the morning when she got out of bed. She read on the Internet that ginger is a good remedy for the "whirls." She stocked up on ginger supplements at her local health-food store and took them for a few weeks. Then one morning she stood up in the bathtub, passed out, and fell and broke her wrist.

She was lucky in a way. The emergency room doctor who treated her took the time to find out why the accident happened in the first place. Ginger is in fact a traditional remedy for vertigo, a type of dizziness often associated with inner-ear disturbances. But Clara didn't have vertigo. What she had was orthostatic hypotension, a sudden drop in blood pressure sometimes caused by too-high doses of blood pressure medicine. Her doctor lowered her dose, and the dizziness went away.

Even though most home remedies are safe, people sometimes take them for the wrong reasons. Or they diagnose themselves when they really need a doctor. Some conditions are easy to recognize and treat at home. You don't need a battery of tests for gums that bleed for a couple of days or for the occasional upset stomach. But it's not always easy to tell what's minor and what's not.

That's one reason it's important to check with your doctor before taking herbs or other supplements, or at least let your doctor know what you're already taking, especially if you're using other medicines at the same time. It's not uncommon for supplements to alter the effects of over-the-counter or prescription drugs—another good reason to be honest with your doctor about what supplements you take. For example, people who take high-dose vitamin E along with blood-thinning drugs have an increased risk of internal bleeding.

Even if a tea or an herb seems completely innocuous, if you're taking it regularly to treat a health problem—stinging nettle for arthritis, for example, or dandelion to lower blood pressure—let your doctor know. Some herbs aren't as effective as people claim, and you don't want to make a mistake and undertreat a potentially serious problem. Even if a supplement is safe and does what the manufacturer says it does, it won't do a bit of good if you take it for a condition you don't actually have—and you could wind up missing a health problem that's too serious to ignore.

Even though most home remedies are safe, people sometimes take them for the wrong reasons.

Proceeding with Some Cautions

If traditional cures have been used daily for thousands of years, they probably work or people wouldn't use them. But there are always risks—of side effects, interactions with drugs, or simply using the wrong remedy. The home remedies in this book are supported by anecdotal evidence of their effectiveness—and in many cases by scientific studies—and they have been carefully screened for safety by our board of medical advisors. But there are times when you'll want to exercise extra caution, such as:

If you are pregnant. Do not take any herbs, supplements, or over-the-counter (OTC) medications without first consulting your doctor. Many of these can affect the health of the fetus, particularly if they are taken in large doses.

If you are taking prescription medication. Talk to your doctor about possible interactions between your prescribed medication and any herbs, supplements, or over-the-counter drugs recommended in this book. The cautions on pages 245–248 provide some guidelines about drug, herb, and supplement interactions and some additional cautions. But you should also tell your doctor about any other supplements or medications that you take at the same time—particularly if you have a chronic condition such as diabetes or heart disease.

If you know you are allergic to a food or medication. Exercise caution or consult your doctor before you eat or drink any remedy that might contain the allergen.

If you have a serious health condition. Pay special attention to "Should I Call the Doctor?" at the beginning of each section. The purpose of these home remedies is to help you deal with everyday ailments and improve your overall health—not to mask serious conditions that require medical treatment.

If you are treating a child or infant. Some herbs, supplements, and home remedies just aren't appropriate for children or babies. Unless a remedy is specifically recommended for children, ask your pediatrician for advice before treating your kids. And choose over-the-counter products designed for children rather than adults (Children's Tylenol, for instance, instead of regular Tylenol).

Herbal Healing

When James A. Duke slipped a disk in his upper back in the early 1990s, he tried all the things his doctor recommended: rest, ultrasound, and stomach-gnawing doses of anti-inflammatory drugs. He didn't stop there. He took licorice to settle his stomach, milk thistle to protect his liver from the aspirin, and echinacea before surgery to protect against infection.

Duke, a former botanist at the U.S. Department of Agriculture, author of *The Green Pharmacy*, and a leading expert on medicinal herbs, is one of millions of people who appreciate the healing powers of nature's plants. In fact, according to the World Health Organization, about 80 percent of the world's population depends on herbs as their primary source of medical care. They're cheaper than drugs, and in many cases, they're just as effective. What's more, they're often safer than drugs.

About 80 percent of the world's population depends on herbs as their primary source of medical care.

When you're used to snapping open a childproof cap and popping a convenient capsule, dealing with dried herbs can be a bit daunting. It shouldn't be. Nearly all herbs are available in capsule or liquid forms, with dosing instructions printed on the label. You can also buy bulk herbs—leaves, seeds, stems, or whatever part of the plant contains the active ingredients—at many health-food stores and brew them into tasty (or not so tasty!) teas.

You can easily grow your own herbs in your garden or in windowsill pots. The usual approach is to snip the stems, rinse the herbs with water to remove any dirt, then hang them upside down to dry. When the leaves feel brittle but aren't so dry that they crumble, pluck them and store them in a dark container. Packing jars to the lid keeps out oxygen and

Grow Your Own: Fresh Herbs Within Reach

You don't have to have a green thumb to grow medicinal herbs. Most thrive with a minimum of care as long as they're planted in good soil and get adequate amounts of sunshine. Here are a few versatile herbs to start with:

ALOE VERA leaves contain a clear gel that kills bacteria and helps cuts and burns heal more quickly. It's among the easiest herbs to grow because it requires little water and no daily care.

Planting tips: Buy a small plant and transfer it to a window planter filled with potting soil. Keep it warm; aloe vera doesn't like temperatures below about 40 degrees. As long as you keep it warm and watered, it will continue to put out new leaves.

How to use: Cut one of the fleshy leaves and squeeze the gel on minor cuts or burns. The gel dries and forms an invisible bandage, keeping bacteria out and moisture in.

CHAMOMILE is among the sweetest-flavored medicinal herbs. It has anti-inflammatory and intestine-soothing chemical compounds, but most people sip chamomile tea to ease anxiety and insomnia.

Planting tips: German chamomile, the most popular form, is an annual. Sow the seeds in the spring after the danger of frost has passed. Scatter the seeds in beds, tamp them down, and keep the soil moist. Chamomile prefers well-drained soil in areas that are partially shaded.

How to use: Snip the stems and hang to dry. Pluck off the dry leaves and store in dark, sealed containers to preserve the medicinal oils.

GARLIC grows in almost any soil, and it's among the most potent herbs in terms of flavor as well as healing. Eating a clove or two daily may help prevent colds, lower cholesterol, inhibit blood clots in the arteries, and reduce the risk of heart disease and stroke.

Planting tips: Break cloves from a head of garlic and plant them in full sun about two inches deep. Keep the soil slightly moist at first, but don't overwater. During summer, cut back the flower stalk so the plant puts all of its energy into producing fat, rich-tasting cloves. Harvest the bulbs in late summer.

How to use: Peel the cloves and add to recipes—or eat them whole if you like the extra-strong taste. Eat one to two cloves daily during the cold season for infection-fighting protection.

LICORICE ROOT has a deliciously sweet taste that's perfect for teas, especially when you're fighting a cold or cough. It contains a chemical compound, glycyrrhizinic acid, that suppresses coughs and soothes sore throats.

Planting tips: Licorice is grown from root cuttings that contain "eyes." Plant the cuttings vertically about an inch deep in rich, well-drained soil. The plants reach three to seven feet and have beautiful purple flowers. The roots can be harvested in the fall after the first year or two.

How to use: Dig up the roots, split them in half, and store them in a dark, shady place to dry; it takes about six months. Powder the root, add about half a teaspoon to a cup of boiling water, and steep for about 10 minutes.

ROSEMARY belongs in the spice cabinet as well as the medicine chest. It contains chemicals that aid digestion, fight bacteria, and act as a mental stimulant.

Planting tips: You can plant rosemary from seed, but cuttings are more likely to thrive. Place them in full sun in sandy soil, with about one-third of the twig showing.

How to use: Strip the leaves and store them in a dark, shady place until dry, then use to make a tasty tea.

helps maintain freshness. If you're using herbs grown for their flowers, harvest the flowers just after the plant blooms.

Most herbal teas call for adding one rounded teaspoon of dried herb (or a tablespoon of fresh) to a cup of boiling water. Steep for about 10 minutes, let cool, then drink. (Teas made from bark, seeds, or roots need to steep longer.) Start with small amounts of tea—say, one to three cups daily. Only use larger amounts under the supervision of a professional herbalist or an herb-friendly doctor.

Other Supplements

"Supplements" used to mean garden-variety vitamins and minerals that people took to give their diets a boost. Today, pharmacy shelves practically sag under the weight of amino acids, natural hormones, and antioxidants, to name just a few.

For a long time, doctors pooh-poohed the sometimes extravagant claims of supplement manufacturers. To be sure, there are a lot of questionable products, with claims ranging from instant weight loss to overnight improvements in virility. On the other hand, even tradition-bound doctors have come to realize that some supplements have earned their place alongside conventional drugs.

Even tradition-bound doctors have come to realize that some supplements have earned their place alongside conventional drugs.

Glucosamine is a good example. It was initially dismissed by the medical community as snake-oil treatment, but studies in the last ten years have shown that it does in fact help the body repair damaged cartilage. Rheumatologists and orthopedists now routinely recommend it to people who need relief from arthritic joints. Maria Garcia, a Santa Fe homemaker, takes it every morning because it keeps her shoulders mobile and pain-free. Just to see what happened, she quit taking glucosamine for a few weeks—and her pain came right back.

Lycopene is another supplement that's received a lot of scientific attention. An antioxidant found in tomatoes and sold in supplement form, it helps lower a man's risk of prostate cancer. Coenzyme Q_{10}, a chemical naturally produced by the body, improves the heart's pumping ability in people with congestive heart failure. Fish-oil capsules may lower levels of cholesterol along with inflammatory chemicals that increase the risk of heart attack. The list goes on and on.

Buying and Using Herbs and Supplements

You don't have to spend more than a few minutes on the Internet to realize that a lot of the claims about supplements are dubious, to say the least. Nutritional supplements are given only cursory attention by the Food and Drug Administration. Manufacturers aren't allowed to promise specific health benefits on the labels, but they can do almost anything else. If you'd like to know more about supplements and what they really do, visit the Web site of the Office of Complementary and Alternative Medicine, part of the National Institutes of Health. There you'll find useful information, including reports of recent clinical studies.

Even if an herb or other supplement has been proven to be safe and effective, there's no guarantee that the particular product you're buying contains the active ingredients in the right amounts. Look to the following advice to help you choose a quality product.

Buy reputable brands. When independent laboratories analyze the contents of supplement bottles, they occasionally find, well, nothing very useful. Supplements may contain little or even none of the advertised active ingredient. And the amounts of those ingredients can vary unpredictably from pill to pill. How can you be sure the brand you're buying is a good one? One place to start is consumerlab.com. There you'll find the results of independent tests on many products.

Choose standardized supplements. Whenever possible, buy supplements with the word "standardized" on the label. This indicates that each pill or capsule contains a specified amount of the active ingredient.

Look for "USP." This stands for United States Pharmacopeia, an independent body of experts that sets standards of purity and potency for vitamins, minerals, and some herbs. A label marked "USP" means the product meets these standards, at least according to the manufacturer. If a label doesn't say "USP," it may be because the USP hasn't set guidelines for that supplement or the manufacturer chose not to perform the necessary tests. But if you have the choice between a product that's labeled "USP" and one that isn't, choose the one that is.

Aromatherapy: The Scents of Healing

As you stroll through an herb garden, it's hard to resist the temptation to pluck a few leaves, crush them between your fingers, and enjoy the rich, pleasant fragrance. We now know those scents are not only pleasant but often therapeutic. Captured in essential oils, the fragrances pass directly to nerve centers of our brain, where they produce a wide range of responses. Essential oils can help relieve anxiety and depression, tame our physical reactions to stress, induce sleep, and enhance energy. Research shows that the scents of certain herbs—such as lavender, bergamot, marjoram, and sandalwood—actually alter brain waves, helping to induce relaxation and sleep.

Essential oils can help relieve anxiety and depression, banish stress, induce sleep, and enhance energy.

Today we can get these benefits from commercially prepared, highly concentrated essential oils. A plant may contain as little as one percent fragrant oil, but when that oil is extracted and distilled, the scent is intense. To make one ounce of Bulgarian rose oil, for example, requires 600 pounds of rose petals. One drop of herbal oil holds the equivalent of two cups of tea.

You can enjoy the healing benefits of essential oils in several different ways—inhaling the fragrance, soaking in water that contains an oil, or massaging it onto your skin. To inhale the fragrance, just put a drop or two of essential oil on a handkerchief or several drops on a lightbulb or lightbulb ring. Or, if you want to be surrounded by the scent, you can purchase a vaporizer or diffuser and follow the directions.

When you're using an oil for bathing or massage, you need to dilute it with a "carrier" oil. To create a massage oil, add 8 to 12 drops of essential oil to 8 teaspoons of a cold-pressed plant oil such as sweet-almond, grape-seed, or sunflower oil. For bathing, the usual mix is 10 to 30 drops of essential oil in 20 teaspoons of an unscented white lotion. Simply add this mix to the bathwater.

Because essential oils are so highly concentrated, they should not be taken internally. Some people have an allergic reaction to oils, so you'll want to take some care when trying out a new oil. Also, since essential oils can pass through the skin into the bloodstream, they should not be used by pregnant women. Talk to a qualified practitioner before applying essential oil if you have sensitive skin, epilepsy, high blood pressure, or if you've recently had an operation.

To make sure you purchase high-quality essential oils and store them properly, you may want to get some advice from an aromatherapist. Many of these oils can be stored for years without losing their fragrance, though some citrus oils—like orange and lemon—need to be refrigerated. Store them in dark bottles, tightly sealed, preferably in a cool place and always away from sunlight.

What Is Homeopathy?

If you haven't encountered homeopathy before, you might be wary of the strange little bottles marked with "C's" and "X's" on the shelves of many health-food stores. But there's no reason to fear these remedies. The homeopathic mixtures recommended in this book are extremely safe, and many of them have won widespread respect as healing agents—even if it's impossible to explain why they work.

Imagine taking a single drop of any drug—say, a liquid decongestant. Dilute that drop with 10 drops of water. Shake the mixture well, take out a single drop, and dilute it with another 10 drops of water. Repeat the process a few times, and what's left? According to the laws of science, not much. But according to homeopathy, the highly diluted mixture is among the most powerful drugs you can take.

You can see why homeopathy, a style of medicine developed by a German physician more than 200 years ago, hasn't won a lot of support in the mainstream medical community. But the experience of millions of Americans—and a handful of scientific studies—suggest there's something to it.

Here are the basics. Working from a list of more than 2,000 substances, homeopaths give sick patients a substance that in large doses would mimic the symptoms caused by their disease—but in very small amounts, theoretically relieves the symptoms. Most of the remedies used in homeopathy come from herbs or minerals. For example, St. John's wort for depression, comfrey for wounds or bruises, and eyebright for tired, burning eyes. But many are diluted with so much water that they contain little or even none of the active ingredient.

Most experts say that homeopathy violates a basic principle of pharmaceutical science: The *smaller* the dose, the *smaller* the effects. Yet researchers who study homeopathy have come up with some intriguing results. A study of 478 flu patients, for example, found that 17 percent of those treated with homeopathy improved, compared to just 10 percent of those taking placebos. The prestigious *British Medical Journal*, in an analysis of 107 scientific studies of homeopathic medicines, found that 77 percent of them showed positive effects.

An analysis of 107 scientific studies of homeopathic medicines found that 77 percent of them showed positive effects.

It's been suggested that the process of diluting and shaking the solutions somehow "potentizes" the remaining water and changes its chemical properties. But no one really knows how—or whether—homeopathy actually works. Since the doses of active ingredients are so small, however, there's no harm in trying it. That's what Gail Robinson of Kansas City, Missouri, thought when she took homeopathic doses of St. John's wort for depression. "I felt better than I had in years," she says.

You can buy homeopathic remedies in health-food stores, but you'll still want to work with an experienced homeopath. Different remedies are used for each symptom you're experiencing—and the remedies as well as the doses may change depending on your mental and emotional state at the time.

The doses used in homeopathy are confusing at first. You'll usually see them listed as X or C on the label. A 1X remedy has been diluted one time, using one part of the active ingredient in 10 parts water. A 2X solution contains one part of the active ingredient in 100 parts water, and a 3X solution contains one part of the active ingredient in 1,000 parts water. The C solutions are even more dilute; they may not contain even a single molecule of the original active ingredient.

Homeopathy isn't a substitute for regular medical care. Most homeopaths spend at least an hour with new patients. They take a complete health history, review your symptoms, and decide whether or not homeopathy is appropriate for you—and whether you need to see a conventional doctor.

Mind-Body Medicine

For many of the health conditions in this book, you'll find a number of remedies that involve meditation, progressive relaxation, yoga, or tai chi. Whatever form they take, relaxation and meditation techniques have proved their power. In recent years, the success of mind-body healing has been borne out by some remarkable evidence.

One of the most well-studied practices is transcendental meditation, or TM. In exploring the benefits of TM, Harvard researcher Herbert Benson, M.D., measured the physical responses of students who would sit quietly with their eyes closed and repeat a word or phrase (called a mantra) over and over again. The twenty-minute "exercises" were done once or twice a day. Dr. Benson discovered that the profound calm induced by TM could lower blood pressure as well as slow heart rate and breathing. Benson termed this the *relaxation response*. Many of the stress-relief benefits of meditation also help increase immunity and combat problems such as anxiety and depression.

Since all kinds of meditation and relaxation techniques can be done at home at any time and with minimal preparation, they are recommended for many health conditions, ranging from anxiety and high blood pressure to psoriasis and menstrual problems.

If you have no experience with meditation, start with a simple twenty-minute exercise that will give you some practice. Just sit in a comfortable, upright position, with your back straight, your head upright, and your body relaxed. With your eyes closed, concentrate completely on your breathing. Take deep, steady breaths, feeling the rise and fall of your abdomen, not your chest. Focus on a word or sound, such as "peace" or "om," and repeat it over and over again. Anytime your attention wanders, bring it back to your word or sound and your breathing again. After about twenty minutes, stop, open your eyes, and stretch. Go slowly at first as you stand up and begin to move around again.

If you find that you have difficulty meditating, you might want to get further guidance from an instructor who practices

TM, yoga, or tai chi. Many classes are offered at health clubs, community centers, or adult-education centers.

You don't necessarily have to practice meditation or deep breathing to elicit the relaxation response. Many religions include practices of regular worship or reflection that can provide similar benefits, Dr. Benson has pointed out. Follow-up research has shown that daily prayer, for example, can help relieve various health problems and even help prolong life.

Teaming Up with Professionals

Even though Americans see non-M.D. health professionals more often than we see primary care physicians and spend billions of dollars a year on herbs and supplements, we obviously haven't given up on conventional medicine. Nor are we interested in substituting one type of medicine for another. What most of us want is the best of both worlds—the cutting-edge tools of modern medicine combined with the natural, at-home treatments that earlier generations depend on.

This approach, known as complementary medicine, makes good sense. If you have heart disease or diabetes, for example, you'll obviously want the most advanced care you can get. Yet there's so much you can do yourself at the same time—not only to relieve symptoms and feel better, but also to give nature a hand and help your body reverse the condition or recover more quickly.

Don't hesitate to talk to your doctor about the remedies you use at home. You may even discover that your doctor has his or her own favorites, like flushing away ear pain with hydrogen peroxide, massaging away a headache, or soothing a rash with an oatmeal bath. After all, conventional medicine and at-home remedies aren't the adversaries they're sometimes made out to be. Each has strengths and weaknesses—and both work best when they're used hand in hand.

If you're especially interested in herbs, acupuncture, and other "natural" healing methods, consider seeing a naturopathic doctor (N.D.). These doctors specialize in treating health problems using a wide range of therapies.

The Remedies: A Final Word

This book contains a huge number of remedies from a wide variety of sources, including traditional folk remedies. Many of the traditional "recipes" we found for teas, elixirs, and tonics called for specific measurements. A grandmother may have specified, for instance, 2 teaspoons of honey, 24 cloves of garlic, or 3 handfuls of pokeberry root. But in many cases the exact amounts aren't critical to the success of the remedy. So the quantities that you find in this book may differ slightly from those in home remedies that you have heard about from your own family.

Complementary medicine is what most of us are looking for. It's the best of both worlds—the cutting-edge advances of modern medicine combined with natural, at-home treatments.

For each "recipe," however, we've included the ingredients that are most likely to provide some direct health benefits, while omitting those that are ineffective or might cause problems.

Whenever possible, we recommend ingredients available from common sources. In some cases, the ingredients in "regional" recipes have been excluded. Health cures used in India and Pakistan, for example, include herbs and spices such as Indian pennywort, butterfly pea, cardamom, cinnamon, cyperus, and turmeric. In this book, we have only included the ones that can be found in most grocery stores. If you can't find a remedy in the grocery store, check your local health-food store or medical supply store. If you still have a hard time finding a product, you may be able to order it online, so try searching the Internet.

Of course, many of the remedies in this book don't require any special supplies at all—just the right food, exercise, or hands-on healing. Temporary relief, or even a cure, may be as near as your kitchen shelf or medicine cabinet.

If one remedy doesn't work for you, try another. If it does work, be sure to tell a loved one or friend so that they might one day benefit from it too. Happy healing!

Acne

If scientists can decipher the human genome, you'd think they could find a way to eradicate acne. No such luck. It's up to you to deal with the outbreaks that can damage your pride of appearance long after teenage angst is past. When a pimple rears its ugly black, white, or red head, over-the-counter products can help. But so can simple remedies from Mother Nature's medicine chest.

What's wrong

Your skin is producing too much sebum—the thick, oily substance that acts as a natural lubricant—and the excess is blocking your pores. There are two kinds of acne. The most common form, acne vulgaris, shows up on your face, chest, shoulders, or back as blackheads, whiteheads, or red blemishes. Cystic acne appears as painful cysts or firm, painless lumps. Fluctuating hormones caused by puberty, menstruation, pregnancy, perimenopause, or birth-control pills often increase the production of sebum, which can trigger an outbreak of either type. Other culprits include emotional stress, clothing that rubs against the skin, and some drugs, such as steroids. Genetics may also play a role.

Zap Zits Now

The first avenue of assault is an over-the-counter cream or gel formulated with **benzoyl peroxide**. It works by mildly irritating the skin, which encourages dying skin cells to flake off. This helps reopen clogged pores. Benzoyl peroxide also kills the bacteria that infect clogged pores.

Alpha-hydroxy acids (AHAs), such as glycolic acid, slough off the outermost layer of skin, which helps keep pores clear and unclogged. Opt for a cream, lotion, or gel that contains 8% glycolic acid.

At the first hint of a pimple, wrap an **ice cube** in a piece of plastic wrap and hold it to the area at least twice a day—every hour, if you can, but for no longer than five minutes each time. The cold will reduce the redness and ease the inflammation.

Pop an **aspirin** or two. Taking one or two 325-milligram tablets four times a day can help calm an acne outbreak by reducing inflammation. (Check with your doctor before taking aspirin regularly.)

Try Alternative Acne Treatments

Three times a day, dab a drop of **tea-tree oil** on blemishes to discourage infection and speed healing. Research has found that 5% tea-tree oil is as effective against acne as a 5% benzoyl peroxide solution.

For acne that flares at that time of the month, drink one to two cups of **chasteberry tea** a day. Some studies show that this herb helps regulate female hormones. Give the herb two or three months to work. And don't drink copious amounts of the tea to hasten the results—it may make your skin look worse.

➤ Dab **vinegar** or **lemon juice** on pimples. All vinegars contain acids that can help flush out pores—so does lemon juice.

➤ An old folk remedy for healing pimples is to use a mixture of **spice and honey** on them. Combine 1 teaspoon powdered nutmeg and 1 teaspoon honey, and apply it to the pimple. Leave on for 20 minutes, then wash off. There's no proof that this helps, but honey does have antiseptic properties.

➤ Apply **aloe vera.** One study found that 90 percent of skin sores were completely healed with aloe vera within five days.

➤ Think **zinc.** People with acne tend to have lower than normal zinc levels. Zinc supplements produce visible improvement in about a third of people who take them. You'll need high doses, though—between 200 and 600 milligrams daily—so take it only under your doctor's supervision.

The Power of Prevention

➤ If you keep skin free of dirt and excess oil—the thinking goes—perhaps your pores will never get clogged. But over-cleansing can cause acne by making your sebaceous glands produce more oil. **Forgo granulated cleansers.** And **avoid washcloths**; they are abrasive and can accumulate bacteria if you reuse them. Instead, use a disposable cleansing cloth.

➤ Make a skin-cleansing solution to help clear up black-heads. Add one teaspoon of **Epsom salt** and three drops of **iodine** to one-half cup of water and bring to a boil. Let cool. Dip in a clean cotton pad and use it to clean the pores.

➤ Men: **Rinse your razor** in alcohol after you use it so any bacteria it harbors won't transfer itself to your face.

Should I call **the doctor?**

Getting a pimple now and then is no big deal. But a visit to a dermatologist is in order if your blemishes don't respond to over-the-counter treatments within three months or your skin becomes severely inflamed, with painful, fluid-filled lumps and a reddish or purplish cast. You'll want a doctor to take a look at your skin if it's always red and flushed, even if acne isn't present; you may have the beginnings of rosacea, a skin condition characterized by persistent redness, pimples, and enlarged blood vessels.

To Squeeze or Not to Squeeze

If you absolutely, positively must squeeze your blemishes, here's the dermatologist-approved method—and it's only valid for whiteheads. Clean the area well. Light a match and hold the tip of a needle in the flame for three seconds. Then gently nick the surface of the pimple. Use a cotton swab to drain it, then clean it with hydrogen peroxide, if you wish. But don't squeeze or pick—you'll make it worse. To "squeeze" a blackhead, use a blackhead extractor, available in drugstores. Soften the blemish with a hot-water compress for 10 minutes before you use it, and wash your hands beforehand to reduce the chances of infection.

Age Spots

Let them count your birthday candles, not your age spots! The best way to block the spots—and skin cancer too—is by slathering on the sunscreen. But if past lapses have shown up on your skin, shop for an over-the-counter fade cream, or raid your kitchen for a simple spot remover. Keep in mind that it may take weeks or months to see improvement. And from this day forward, vow never to leave the house without proper protection.

What's wrong

Despite their name, these flat or rounded brown spots that dot the backs of your hands or face aren't caused by age. They're simply areas of excess pigment, which result from years of unprotected sun exposure. Because it takes decades to see the sun damage, many people won't notice the splotches until later in life, but people who have had significant sun exposure can develop them in their 20s and 30s. Some drugs can make you more vulnerable to sun damage and related age spots, including tetracycline, diuretics (water pills), and drugs for diabetes and blood pressure.

Lighten Up

➤ A fade cream called **Porcelana** contains a 2% solution of the bleaching agent hydroquinone. (Darker spots may need a 3% solution, but for that you will need a prescription from a dermatologist.) Before you use Porcelana, read the package directions.

➤ Dab the juice of a fresh **lemon** on the spots at least twice a day. Lemon juice is mildly acidic, and may be strong enough to slough off the skin's outer layer and remove or lighten age spots.

➤ Blend **honey and yogurt** to create a natural bleach that can lighten age spots. Mix 1 teaspoon of plain yogurt and 1 teaspoon of honey. Apply, let dry for 30 minutes, then rinse. Do this once a day.

➤ Spread your spots with **aloe vera gel**, straight from the leaves of a living plant, if possible. The plant contains chemicals that slough away dead cells and encourages the growth of new, healthy ones. Apply the gel once or twice a day.

➤ Try **buttermilk**. An old folk remedy for age spots, it contains lactic acid, which gently exfoliates sun-damaged skin and pigmented areas.

Go Undercover

➤ Camouflage age spots with a cosmetic concealer like **Dermablend**, a heavy foundation sold at major department stores. Ask a salesperson to help you pick the right shade for your skin and show you how to apply it.

The Power of Prevention

⚬ **Avoid the sun** as much as possible during peak hours—10 A.M. to 4 P.M. during summer, and 10 A.M. to 2 P.M. in the winter.

⚬ Every day, 30 minutes before you set foot outside, slather your skin—including your face and the backs of your hands—with **sunscreen**. Make sure it has a sun protection factor (SPF) of at least 15. The most effective sunscreens for guarding against age spots contain zinc oxide or titanium dioxide. If you will be outdoors for long periods of time, reapply every two hours.

⚬ To help prevent sun rays from penetrating your clothing, try the product called **Rit Sun Guard**. Added to your laundry during the wash cycle, it boosts the SPF of your clothing and prevents 96 percent of the sun's ultraviolet waves from reaching your skin.

⚬ After you've been out in the sun, slather on some **vitamin E** oil. An antioxidant, vitamin E may help prevent age spots by neutralizing skin-damaging free radical molecules. Because vitamin E produces free radicals when it's exposed to sunlight, smooth it on only *after* sun exposure.

Should I call **the doctor?**

Age spots, which usually look like dark, smooth freckles, are generally harmless. However, if a spot starts to tingle, itch, change size or color, or bleed, it's time to call the doctor. Some skin cancers, like melanoma, can look like age spots. If home remedies don't work on your age spots, your dermatologist can most likely get rid of them through laser treatment or by applying liquid nitrogen.

Allergies

Itchy, scratchy, sneezy—they might sound like three of the Seven Dwarfs, but in fact they're allergy symptoms that can leave you, well, grumpy. Reach for an allergy pill if you wish—take it *before* an allergy attack sets in for better results—or try one of the natural antihistamines listed below. You'll also want to wage war on pollen, mites, dander, and other microscopic menaces that send your immune system into overdrive.

What's **wrong**

Allergies? Your symptoms are signs that your immune system is on a rampage, reacting to normally harmless substances like pollen, ragweed, dust, pet dander, or mold. Usually, the immune system ignores these "triggers" and concentrates on protecting you from real threats, such as viruses or bacteria. But when you have allergies, your immune system can't tell certain benign substances from dangerous ones. Triggers can include substances you eat (such as wheat and peanuts), absorb through the skin (such as poison ivy or insect venom), inhale (such as mold or dander), or receive by injection (such as a shot of penicillin).

Nature's Antihistamines

Nettle contains a substance that works as a natural antihistamine. In fact, the famous naturopathic doctor Andrew Weil reportedly takes it for his allergies. You'll find capsules of the freeze-dried leaf in health-food stores. Take 500 milligrams three times a day.

Ginkgo biloba has become renowned for its memory-boosting properties, but it can also be an effective allergy fighter. Ginkgo contains substances called ginkgolides, which can stop certain allergy-triggering chemicals (platelet activating factor, or PAF) in their tracks. Take 60 to 240 milligrams a day.

Quercetin, the pigment that gives grapes their purple hue and puts the green in green tea, inhibits the release of histamine. Take one 500-milligram capsule twice a day. (*Off-limits* . . . if you're already taking nettle, which contains quercetin.)

Try Something Fishy

Omega-3 fatty acids help counter inflammatory responses in the body, such as those triggered by allergies. Salmon and mackerel are good sources of these fats. If you prefer the idea of fish-oil capsules, try taking 3,000 milligrams a day.

Flaxseeds are another excellent source of omega-3 fatty acids. Take one tablespoon of flaxseed oil a day. You can add it to a glass of juice or blend it into a smoothie, but avoid heating it.

Use a Simple Soother

🍃 To soothe red, itchy, swollen eyes, dampen a washcloth with **cool water** and place it over your eyes. Repeat as often as necessary.

🍃 **Saline nasal sprays** are time-tested mucus-busters and can also help to keep your nasal passages moisturized. However, a recent study shows that some commercially made sprays contain a preservative that can actually damage the cells of your sinuses, so it may be safer to make your own. Dissolve a half-teaspoon salt in eight ounces warm water. Load a bulb syringe, lean over the sink, and spritz the saline into your nose.

Repel Pollen Attacks

🍃 **Stay indoors** with the windows closed and the air conditioner turned on to filter out pollen, especially in the early evening, when pollen counts hit their peak.

🍃 **Take shelter** inside before a **thunderstorm**—and up to three hours afterward. Storms are preceded by high humidity, which makes pollen grains swell, burst, and release their irritating starch.

🍃 When you have to go out, wear **wraparound sunglasses** to keep the pollen away from your eyes. And if you don't mind resembling Michael Jackson, a face mask works well too.

🍃 You can also protect yourself outdoors with a "pollen trap." Dab a little **petroleum jelly** under your nose—trap spores that are wafting around before they land in your nostrils.

🍃 When you're in a car, keep the **windows closed**. Turn on the air conditioner to filter out the pollen, and choose the "recirculate" setting so you don't pull in pollinated air.

🍃 **Wash your hair** prior to going to bed so you don't transmit a headful of dust and pollen to your pillow.

Should I call **the doctor?**

Allergic symptoms run the gamut from the merely miserable to the downright dangerous. If drugstore remedies don't do the trick or no longer work, or you can't figure out what you're allergic to, it's time to call the doctor. Wheezing or difficulty breathing requires an immediate call: It can be a sign of an asthma attack or other serious allergic reaction. Ditto if you develop hives or welts. Hives may signal the onset of a potentially fatal allergic reaction—for example, to a bee sting.

Love to Garden? Don't Throw In the Trowel

Most ornamental flowering plants don't release pollen—they rely on insects to pollinate them. Generally speaking, the plants that release the most pollen are trees, grasses, and ragweed. So put on your gardening gloves, and continue to prune those prizewinning roses. Daisies and chrysanthemums are fine too.

Solve a Mighty Problem

🙠 **Dust mites,** nasty little flesh-eating monsters too small to be seen by the naked eye, live in your carpets, curtains, and bedding. Their feces can be a significant cause of allergies. To starve mites of the dust they eat—which is made of your skin—**cover your mattress, box spring, and pillows** with covers made specifically to repel allergens. These covers are sold in drugstores and department stores.

🙠 **Vacuum your carpets** regularly. If you can afford one, purchase a vacuum cleaner that uses a double bag and a HEPA (high-efficiency particulate-arresting) filter. These machines can filter out allergens that are microscopic in size. If you have attractive flooring underneath your carpets, think about getting rid of the carpets altogether.

🙠 **Change your sheets** once a week and wash them in very hot water to kill the mites.

🙠 **Clear away clutter,** which can house mites.

🙠 If you don't have **a dehumidifier,** it's a good idea to get one. Keeping the air in your home dry will significantly reduce the population of dust mites, which perish at humidity levels below 45 percent.

Reduce Reactions to Rover and Fluffy

🙠 **Keep your pet out of the bedroom.** Animals' dander, hair, and saliva—all of which linger even when the animal leaves the room—can contribute to allergic reactions.

🙠 Some dogs are perfectly happy in the traditional outdoor

Skip it!

Though air purifiers may seem like a good idea, research has shown that most of them have little effect on allergens. Small machines simply don't have enough power to rid the air of dust and pollen. Electrostatic precipitators, which give particles an electrical charge and use polarized metal plates to pull them out of the air, can actually aggravate allergy symptoms by polluting the indoor air with ozone. There is one type of purifier that is effective, however: those that use HEPA filters.

A Kiss Is Just a Kiss?

Avoiding known food or drug allergens would seem to be easy, but sometimes you can be exposed in not-so-obvious ways. A recent report from the Mayo Clinic describes a woman who had a life-threatening allergic reaction to shellfish when she kissed her boyfriend. He had eaten a few shrimp with dinner an hour before he kissed her good night. Almost immediately, her lips swelled, her throat began to close, she started wheezing, hives appeared, her stomach cramped, and her blood pressure plummeted. Fortunately, she survived. The lesson, however, is clear: If your love partner is allergic to some food, you'll have to give it up as well. No one knows whether simply brushing your teeth or rinsing your mouth out would do much good, so it's better not to take the chance at all.

A Military Maneuver Against Allergies

Allergic to pollen? Try this remedy, tested by the U.S. Army and deemed effective: Eat honey made in your area, and chew the beeswax it comes in. The theory is that by eating honey produced by local bees, you can desensitize your immune system to the local pollen. Starting two months before hay fever season, eat 2 tablespoons of the honey a day, and chew the beeswax for 5 to 10 minutes. Continue until the season is over. While local honey works best, you can give store-bought a try.

doghouse. If you're allergic to yours, that **outdoor lodging** might be the best solution for both of you.

 Give your pet a bath once a week. Bathing can remove up to 85 percent of pet dander. You can use a pet shampoo, grooming solution, or even plain water.

Clear the Air

 The single best thing you can do to keep allergens out of the air is **air-condition** your house. It keeps humidity low, which discourages mold and dust mites, and it filters the air while it cools it. Keep all windows closed when you're running the AC. And be sure to clean the filters at least once a month.

 If you can afford to **install an air filter**, it can bring dramatic relief from allergies to mold, pollen, and pet dander. HEPA filters are best. When you use a HEPA filter in your bedroom, keep the door closed, so it will effectively filter just the air in that room.

 Studies show that vigorous household cleaning significantly reduces dust, mold, dander, and other common allergens. So **do a serious cleaning job** in your home twice a year—once in the spring, and again in the fall. Wash—with bleach—every scrubbable surface, from the insides of cupboards to the baseboards. Clean furniture with a damp cloth. If your allergies are bad, you may want to hire someone to do the cleaning.

 A basement is prime breeding ground for molds, mildew, and dust mites, especially if it gets wet after rainstorms. In any damp basement, **run a dehumidifier** all the time.

 A clothes dryer can spew out all kinds of fine particles of lint and dust. **Make sure the dryer hose is completely sealed,** so that you don't have those allergy-inducers floating through the house.

Angina

As soon as you describe an angina episode to the doctor, he or she is likely to hand you a prescription for a very convenient medication, nitroglycerin. Far from causing an explosion, when used as directed, the pills will help you deal with the onset of attacks, easing the pain and tightness in your chest by getting more blood and oxygen to the heart. As with traveler's checks, you should never leave home without them. But there are plenty of other things you can do to deal with these episodes and even prevent them from happening.

What's wrong

That crushing, squeezing chest pain is telling you—loudly—that your heart isn't getting enough oxygen-rich blood. Most likely, that's because a buildup of a fatty substance called plaque is blocking the arteries that serve the heart. Angina pain often begins below the breastbone and radiates to the shoulder, arm, or jaw. It may be accompanied by shortness of breath, lightheadedness, irregular heartbeat, and anxiety.

Immediate Measures

➤ If you're standing, walking around, or exercising when an attack occurs, **sit down and rest** for a few minutes.

➤ If you're lying down or resting when the telltale pressure presents itself, **change your body position** by sitting or standing up. That takes pressure off the nerve in your heart that is signaling pain. Angina that occurs at rest is a sign that you may be at much higher risk for a heart attack, so call your doctor immediately.

➤ If the attack comes on when you're emotionally excited or anxious, try to **calm yourself.** Like physical stress, mental stress can increase your heart's demand for oxygen. Do your heart a favor by learning yoga, tai chi, meditation, or some other stress-relieving technique you can practice regularly.

Help Your Heart with Supplements

Coenzyme Q_{10} (CoQ_{10}) is a substance that is present in every cell of the body, where it aids in the production of energy. However, 75 percent of people who have angina also have a CoQ_{10} deficiency, so taking supplements may be helpful. In one study, CoQ_{10} supplements cut the frequency of angina attacks in half. People who took it were also able to exercise longer and harder. The usual dose is 150 milligrams twice a day.

Unstop Those Bottled-Up Feelings

Many doctors believe that suppressing your emotions can damage your heart. In studies, men and women who kept their feelings to themselves secreted more of the stress hormone cortisol. Researchers concluded that people who tended to keep their feelings "bottled up" were putting extra stress on the heart. If you can talk to a partner, friend, or counselor about your feelings, instead of trying to keep a stiff upper lip, you may literally help relieve some "heartache."

⬥ **L-carnitine,** an amino acid, helps the heart muscle use its limited oxygen supply more efficiently. In studies, people with angina who took the supplement showed significant improvement in their ability to exercise after 45 weeks. The usual dose is 500 to 1,000 milligrams three times a day.

⬥ Try taking 500 milligrams a day of **hawthorn,** an herb that's been used for heart trouble for more than a century. Hawthorn increases the flow of blood—and thus oxygen—to the heart by dilating blood vessels. It may also increase the force of heart contractions.

The Power of Prevention

⬥ With your doctor's help, develop a program of moderate physical **exercise,** which can help ward off angina pain.

⬥ **If you smoke, quit.** The nicotine in cigarettes constricts the arteries, triggering angina or making it worse.

⬥ If you're a java junkie, keep your habit in check. Research shows that drinking five or more cups of **coffee** a day can increase your risk for angina attacks.

⬥ After eating a large or heavy meal, rest or **engage in some quiet activity** like reading. When you have a big meal, the body diverts extra blood flow to the digestive tract to aid digestion, meaning the heart receives less oxygen and is more vulnerable to an attack.

⬥ **Don't stay out in cold weather.** Cold air stimulates muscular reflexes that can cause angina.

⬥ **Avoid sudden physical exertion,** such as running to catch a bus or lifting a heavy object.

Should I call
the doctor?

Many people who experience angina for the first time think they're having a heart attack. While angina does not completely block the flow of blood to the heart, as a heart attack does, it's a warning that should not be ignored. If you think you might have angina, get to the doctor as soon as possible. If you have chest pain, as opposed to chest pressure, that lasts for 15 minutes or is accompanied by shortness of breath and nausea, go to the ER immediately.

Anxiety

If it seems like the causes of your anxiety are all around you, take heart: so are the cures. Herbs and oils to boost the soothing powers of a warm bath, worry-taming teas, and even some classic comfort foods...For those times you're feeling anxious, here are some forms of kindness you owe yourself.

What's wrong

Anxiety is a reaction to a threat or danger that is vague or even unknown. You feel worried, but you're not quite sure why. It can manifest any number of symptoms: poor concentration, sweating, trembling, irritability, rapid heart rate, shallow breathing, or unwanted thoughts or behaviors.

Soak Away Your Cares

A **warm bath** is one of the most pleasant and reliable ways to soothe your senses. For an even better balm, add some **lavender oil** (or dried flowers if you have them) to the tub and soak to your heart's content. Although no one knows what gives this wonderfully scented herb its calming effect, lavender has a 2,000-year-old reputation as a calmative that soothes the nerves. No time for a bath? Dab a bit of lavender oil on your temples and forehead and sit quietly for a few minutes.

Suck It In...Deeply

Regulating your breath can help bring your anxiety under quick control. To slow and deepen your breathing, sit down, put one hand over your abdomen, and slowly inhale so that your belly expands under your hand but your shoulders do not rise. Hold your breath for four or five seconds, then very slowly exhale. Repeat until you feel calmer.

Sip Your Way to Serenity

An old-time remedy for insomnia, drinking a glass of **warm milk**, can tame tension any time of day. Milk contains tryptophan, an amino acid that is needed for the production of the brain chemical serotonin, which enhances feelings of well-being.

Catnip, the dried herb that makes cats bizarrely hyperactive, has the opposite effect on humans. It contains chemicals that act as a mild sedative. Simply purchase catnip tea bags and enjoy a cup as often as you like.

⤙ **Hops**, which give beer its distinctive bitter flavor, have a long history as a sedative. In fact, workers who picked hops in the fields were known to suffer from unexplained sleepiness known as hop-picker fatigue. Place 2 teaspoons of the dried herb in a cup of very hot water. Drink up to three cups of this "anti-anxiety tea" a day.

Don't Fuel the Jitter Bug

⤙ Limit yourself to a single cup of **coffee, tea,** or **cola drink** per day. Studies suggest that people with anxiety symptoms may be more sensitive to caffeine than most people.

⤙ **Watch your intake** of wine, beer, and other alcoholic drinks. While they seem to subdue anxiety at first, when the alcohol wears off, anxiety can actually heighten.

Speed Up and Slow Down

⤙ **Aerobic exercise** is a great anxiety reliever. Taking a brisk 30-minute walk spurs the release of endorphins, chemicals that block pain and improve your mood.

⤙ Whether it's meditating, praying, tending your flowers, or watching your goldfish, do some sort of **meditative activity** for 15 minutes several times a day. Deeply focusing your attention on the moment at hand steers your mind away from anxious thoughts.

Try a Tablet of Tension Tamer

⤙ A pleasant smell *isn't* something you can expect from the herb **valerian**, but if you want relief from anxiety, you might forgive the odor. Research suggests that the active ingredients

Should I call **the doctor?**

Prolonged, severe anxiety can take a serious toll on your physical health. Seek help if you're anxious most of the time, can't sleep or concentrate, turn to alcohol, drugs, or food to quell your anxiety, or feel you might harm yourself or others. It's worth noting that anxiety symptoms can mimic those of serious conditions, such as hyperthyroidism, hypoglycemia, and heart attack, or occur as a side effect of some medications. So it's wise to discuss your symptoms with a doctor.

Anxiety Attacks

Unlike generalized anxiety, anxiety attacks come on suddenly and with overwhelming force. Your heart begins to race, your blood pressure rises, you struggle to breathe, and you feel as if you're about to faint. You may even think you're having a heart attack. Anxiety attacks are most likely to appear after a period of unusual stress, such as a death or divorce. The best way to handle them is to see them for what they are: harmless, if frightening, emotional states. Just tell yourself that you're not in any danger; you're having a panic attack, and it will soon end. Stay calm, try to take a few deep breaths, and let the attack run its course.

Repeat these gut-steeling statements to yourself when facing a situation that threatens to send your anxiety level soaring.

Meeting strangers: "This will be a great opportunity to get to know someone I've never met before."

Beginning a new job: "I am well prepared to begin this job, and I know I will be able to master the skills that will allow me to excel."

Making a public speech or presentation: "I have something important to say that will touch the lives and influence the decisions of everyone in this room."

Initiating a new project: "I will succeed by helping others to be successful and by making my best personal contribution."

Dealing with setbacks and insecurity: "Because I have overcome obstacles like this in the past, I know I will be able to do it again."

When challenged: "It does not matter whether others see me as right or wrong as long as I make the best judgment I can and express my views honestly."

When faced with rejection: "I have been given a terrific opportunity to try new alternatives and take a different path, and I am prepared for new challenges."

in valerian attach to the same receptors in the brain that are affected by the anti-anxiety drug Valium. Take 250 milligrams twice a day and 250 to 500 milligrams before bedtime.

5-hydroxytryptophan (5-HTP) can replenish your supply of serotonin, an anxiety-calming brain chemical. The 5-HTP in your body comes from the amino acid tryptophan, but small quantities are also found in the seeds of griffonia, a tree grown mostly in Ghana and the Ivory Coast. Supplements of 5-HTP are made from extract of the Griffonia or produced synthetically. Take 50 milligrams three times daily with meals. But consult your doctor if you're also taking an antidepressant such as Prozac, Paxil, or Zoloft. These drugs also affect serotonin receptors, and the combined effect could be dangerous.

Swallow a **B-complex multivitamin** each day. Studies show that the B's are natural stress-reducers—the body requires vitamin B_6 to make serotonin, for example—and not getting enough of them can contribute to anxiety.

Arthritis

J oin the club. So many people have osteoarthritis, you'll soon be getting advice not only from your doctor and friends but also from Mom, the plumber, and the next-door neighbor. Yes, anti-inflammatory drugs—prescription and over-the-counter—can ease your pain, and most people will want to take them. But relief doesn't end there. A host of other feel-good, stay-well measures can move you further down the field toward your goal of easy-moving, pain-free days.

Pain Removers

❧ Supplement with **glucosamine** and **chondroitin** to reduce pain and slow cartilage loss. There's evidence that this combination can be effective for people with mild to moderate arthritis. Follow the dosage directions on the label. And keep at it: You might have to use it for a month or more before you begin to see benefits.

❧ Take a half-teaspoon of **powdered ginger** or up to an ounce (about 6 teaspoons) of fresh ginger once a day. Research shows that ginger helps relieve arthritis pain, probably because of its ability to increase blood circulation, which ferries inflammatory chemicals away from painful joints.

❧ Take two 400-milligram doses of **SAM-e** every day. SAM-e has been shown to help relieve arthritis pain by increasing blood levels of proteoglycans—molecules that seem to play a key role in preserving cartilage by helping to keep it "plumped up" and well oxygenated. In a review of SAM-e studies sponsored by the U.S. government, the supplement proved comparable to anti-inflammatory drugs (such as ibuprofen) in fighting arthritis pain. If you get good results with 800 milligrams a day, reduce the dose to 400 milligrams a day after two weeks. If not, you can raise the dose, but don't take more than 1,600 milligrams a day. SAM-e has no known side effects, and it seems to be safe in combination with all prescription and OTC drugs.

What's **wrong**

Of the more than 100 types of arthritis, the most common is osteoarthritis. Symptoms include painfully stiff, swollen joints in any part of the body. The pain is the result of wear and tear on cartilage, the gel-like shock-absorbing material between joints. When cartilage wears away, bone grinds against bone. Although you can develop osteoarthritis at any age, it usually occurs in people over 45, and it's more common among women. Other forms of the disease are rheumatoid arthritis and fibromyalgia.

Should I call **the doctor?**

Since you can't be sure what kind of arthritis you have, or whether your symptoms suggest another condition entirely, report any joint stiffness, swelling, redness, or pain. If you've already been diagnosed with arthritis, call your doctor if you notice a new or different type of swelling in your joints.

Seek Heat Relief and Cold Comfort

✎ **Applying heat** to a painful joint can provide significant relief. For heat sources, you can use electric blankets and mitts, heating pads, or hot packs. Heat things up for 20 minutes. Simply taking a hot bath or shower can also be soothing.

✎ **Cold treatments** may work equally well when joints are inflamed. Wrap an ice cube in a towel or washcloth, and press it to the sore joint. Alternatively, you can use a bag of frozen peas or corn.

Go Hand in Glove to Bed

✎ If you frequently have stiff, swollen hands in the morning, **wear a snug-fitting pair of gloves**, like Isotoners, to bed. They'll keep the swelling in check.

Oil Aching Joints

✎ Eat more **cold-water fish.** Many people who supplement their diets with omega-3 fatty acids—found in cold-water fish like salmon—discover that pain and stiffness are lessened. These substances seem to discourage inflammation in the body.

✎ If you dislike fish, get the healing oils in capsule form. The recommended dose is 2,000 milligrams of an omega-3 supplement three times daily. If you take blood-thinning drugs, check with your doctor before taking **fish-oil capsules.**

✎ As an alternative to fish-oil capsules, take one tablespoon of **flaxseed oil** a day. It's loaded with the same type of omega-3's. Take the oil straight, or add it to your salad dressing.

✎ If you like **nuts**, indulge in them a bit. They also contain beneficial oil.

Rub On Relief

✎ **Capsaicin** is a substance that gives hot peppers their "heat." Rub on a store-bought capsaicin cream (brand names include Zostrix and Capzasin-P) and let it go to work. It irritates nerve endings, diverting your brain's attention from arthritis pain. Capsaicin may also take away pain by depleting the nerves of substance P, a chemical that transmits pain impulses to the brain. You'll need to use it for at least a week or two for full effect.

Rheumatoid Arthritis

A more serious form of arthritis, rheumatoid arthritis, results when the immune system attacks rather than defends the body. Along with joint pain and swelling, rheumatoid arthritis can cause fatigue, poor circulation, anemia, and eye problems. Here are some strategies to cope with the condition:

Start a food diary to track what you were eating when your symptoms flared. You may find that your body's inflammatory response goes into overdrive when you eat wheat, dairy foods, citrus, corn, eggs, or tomatoes.

Try going vegetarian. In a year-long study, people with rheumatoid arthritis who followed a vegetarian diet that was also free of eggs, gluten (a protein in wheat), caffeine, alcohol, salt, refined sugar, and milk products had less pain and swelling in their joints after just one month. And they were able to start eating dairy products again after the first three months or so without any adverse effects.

One study found that people with rheumatoid arthritis who took capsules of gamma-linolenic acid (GLA), the active compound in evening primrose oil, had less pain and inflammation at six months than people who took a placebo. Take 1,000 milligrams of evening primrose oil three times a day.

Some doctors believe that people with rheumatoid arthritis can ease their pain with a brief fast of one or two days. The theory behind fasting is that it gives the overworked immune system a much-needed rest. But check with your doctor before you fast, especially if you take prescription medications.

Oil of wintergreen and **eucalyptus oil** are also effective. Put a few drops on the skin and rub it in. Be cautious with wintergreen, however, since some people develop a skin reaction. Also, don't use either of these oils under a heating pad or hot compress, as the additional heat can cause them to burn or irritate the skin.

Keep Those Joints in Motion

Whether it's walking, swimming, biking, or yoga, commit to a gentle **exercise regimen.** The better your physical condition, the less pain and stiffness you'll have. If you have arthritis in your ankle, knee, or hip, you might need to walk with a cane—at least at first—to help stabilize those joints. If your joints are swollen and inflamed, don't work through the pain. Instead, take a day off.

Talk to your doctor about how to start a **weight-training** program. Strong muscles will help to support your joints and absorb shock.

Tried...

People with arthritis have long worn copper bracelets to "draw out the pain."

...and true

Researchers in Australia have found that people who wear copper bracelets and also take aspirin experience less pain than people who treat their pain with just aspirin.

Try to Measure Up

꙳ If you have hip or knee arthritis, ask your doctor to **measure the length of your legs.** One out of five people with arthritis in these joints has one leg that is slightly longer than the other. Your doctor may be able to suggest corrective shoes for you.

Check the Weather Report

꙳ Many people with arthritis find that their pain is triggered by **changes in the weather.** If you're one of them, it's not all in your head: A sudden increase in humidity and rapid drop in air pressure affect blood flow to arthritic joints. When a storm is brewing, turn on your air conditioner or dehumidifier to dry out the air.

The Power of Prevention

꙳ **Maintain a healthy weight** to help prevent osteoarthritis of the knees and other weight-bearing joints. If you lose just 10 pounds and keep it off for 10 years, you can slash your risk of arthritis in your knees by half, no matter what your current weight.

꙳ If walking is part of your exercise program, make sure you **don't cover the same terrain every day.** Varying the kind of ground you walk on will prevent you from repeatedly stressing the same joints in the same way.

꙳ Invest in a pair of **walking shoes.** The softer heels will lessen the impact of walking on your foot, ankle, leg, and hip joints. Needless to say, high heels are out.

꙳ Recent clinical studies have shown that **vitamin C** and other antioxidants can help reduce the risk of osteoarthritis and its progression. Antioxidants prevent bone breakdown by destroying free radicals—harmful oxygen molecules that cause tissue damage. Take 500 milligrams of vitamin C every day.

꙳ Take **zinc** supplements. One long-term study of nearly 30,000 women found that those who took zinc supplements lowered their risk of rheumatoid arthritis. Taking too much zinc may cause other health risks, however, so limit your intake to one daily 15-milligram dose, and take it with food.

Asthma

For severe asthma attacks—the kind of tightness, wheezing, and shortness of breath that can be really frightening—most people do just what the doctor recommends. Often, that means quick action with an inhaler containing a drug such as albuterol. If that's what you use, and it works, don't give it up. And always have your doctor's telephone number near at hand in case of severe attacks. But for non-emergencies, you'll want to figure out ways to help yourself breathe easy.

Breathe Easier Right Now

When an asthma attack comes on, **stay calm.** Panic can make your symptoms worse. Help yourself along with this visualization trick: Close your eyes. As you inhale, see your lungs expand and fill with white light, and feel your breathing become easier. Repeat this exercise twice more, then open your eyes.

In a pinch, have a strong cup of **coffee** or two 12-ounce bottles of caffeinated cola or Mountain Dew (which is also high in caffeine). Caffeine is chemically related to theophylline, a standard medication for asthma. It helps open airways.

Cancel Your Constriction

Practitioners of traditional Chinese medicine have been using the herb **ginkgo** to treat asthma for centuries. If you want to try it, take 60 to 250 milligrams of standardized ginkgo extract once a day. One recent study suggests that this herb interferes with a protein in the blood that contributes to airway spasms.

Magnesium may make you feel better. Much research suggests that magnesium relaxes the smooth muscles of the upper respiratory tract. The recommended dose is 600 milligrams a day.

Trump Inflammation

Omega-3 fatty acids, found in fatty fish such as tuna, salmon, and mackerel, work much like a class of asthma drugs

What's wrong?

An asthma attack can occur when an irritant—usually a common substance like smoke, cold or dry air, pollen, mold, or dust mites—meets a set of temperamental lungs. Hormonal fluctuations, stress, and anger can also trigger an attack. Sometimes there's no apparent cause. Your difficulty in breathing occurs because the bronchi, the tubes that allow oxygen into your lungs, go into spasms. Accompanying them may be coughing and tightness in the chest. The spasms trigger the release of histamine and other chemicals that cause inflammation and the production of airway-clogging mucus.

Should I call
the doctor?

Yes, if you develop asthma symptoms for the first time. If you're already being treated for asthma, you probably have medication that you take at the onset of an episode. Even so, call your doctor if you notice you're using your medication more often, or if your symptoms worsen even after you take it. Get someone to take you to the emergency room if you can't speak without gasping for breath, develop a bluish cast to your face or lips, find it extremely difficult to breathe, or become confused or exhausted.

called leukotriene inhibitors. These drugs stop the actions of body compounds that cause inflammation in the airways. Take six 1,000-milligram capsules a day in divided doses.

↝ **Evening primrose oil** is rich in an essential fatty acid called GLA, which is converted by the body into anti-inflammatory substances. Take two 500-milligram capsules three times a day. Take them with meals to avoid stomach upset.

↝ **Bioflavonoids**, the compounds that give fruits and vegetables their Technicolor hues, have powerful anti-inflammatory and anti-allergenic properties. One of the best-known bioflavonoids, **quercetin**, inhibits the release of histamine. Take 500 milligrams of quercetin three times a day, 20 minutes before meals.

↝ **Turmeric**, that yellow cooking spice used to flavor Indian curry dishes, is a first-rate anti-inflammatory. The compounds it contains inhibit the release of COX-2 prostaglandins, hormone-like substances involved in inflammation. Mix one teaspoon of turmeric powder in a cup of warm milk and drink this up to three times a day. Turmeric capsules and tinctures are also available.

Keep a Record

↝ In a date book, **make a note of everything you eat** for a month. Also record your asthma symptoms. While food allergies are rarely associated with asthma, occasionally there is a connection. Check your diary against your symptoms to see if anything you're eating increases the frequency or severity of your attacks.

↝ If you take asthma medication, **get a peak-flow meter**, available at drugstores. This gadget measures the speed at which air leaves your lungs—an indication of how well you're breathing. By reading your "peak flow" at certain times, you can tell how well a medication or remedy is working. You can also use it during an attack to determine its severity and decide whether you need emergency care.

The Power of Prevention

↝ **Don't smoke**, and stay away from people who do. Cigarette smoke irritates the airways.

Breathe by the Book

This simple deep-breathing trick can help reduce the severity and frequency of your asthma attacks. When an attack starts, you naturally become more anxious as it gets harder to breathe. This produces a "clenching" response that can further restrict your airways. But if you've practiced this breathing technique ahead of time, you can use it to help yourself breathe more freely.

- Lie on your back on a carpet or mat and place a book on your stomach.

- Inhale gently and deeply, but not by expanding your chest. Instead, expand your abdomen. Keep an eye on the book. If it rises up, you're breathing the right way.

- Just when you think you've reached full capacity, take in a little more air. See if you can raise the book a little higher.

- Exhale gradually, slowly counting to five. The more you exhale, the more relaxed you'll feel.

- Repeat at least five times.

- Don't huddle around a **fireplace** or wood-burning stove.

- In cold weather, **wrap a scarf** around your nose and mouth to help warm frigid air before you inhale it.

- **Be alert** for unusual asthma triggers, such as **strong-scented foods** or the **intensely perfumed sample strips** bound into magazines, and do what you can to avoid them.

- **Try eating smaller, more frequent meals**, and don't eat before you go to bed. The upward migration of stomach acids that cause heartburn can also trigger asthma attacks.

- About 5 percent of people with asthma are allergic to nonsteroidal anti-inflammatory drugs (NSAIDs) like aspirin and ibuprofen. For these people, taking the drugs can trigger an attack. If you are one of them, use an **aspirin-free pain reliever** like acetaminophen (Tylenol) instead.

Athlete's Foot

It's not fair that a locker-room problem should follow you home, but once it does, you have to get tough with it. Consistency counts. Think marathon training, and go the extra mile. The more you can treat your feet and dry your toes, the better. Use these remedies to soothe the itch and fight the fungus that causes it. And follow our prevention tips so athlete's foot doesn't gain a foothold again.

What's wrong

Your feet have been attacked by tinea pedis. This stealthy intruder, which targets the nails, skin, and hair, causes skin to redden, crack, burn, scale, and itch. When the fungus invades the area between your toes, the classic symptom is itchy, flaking skin. Sometimes tinea stays between the toes. But it may also appear on the soles and sides of the feet and even spread to your toenails. Severe cases of athlete's foot can be accompanied by oozing blisters. The locker-room floor is one place where tinea hangs out, but it also loves warm, moist places. Your feet, often confined in sweaty shoes and socks, are an ideal breeding ground.

Bring Itchy Dogs to Heal

When you scan the pharmacy shelves for an OTC remedy, look for creams and ointments that contain **miconazole nitrate** or **tolnaftate.** Massage a small amount into the affected area two or three times a day. And don't make the mistake of stopping the cream when your symptoms subside. Use it for six weeks or more to permanently eradicate the fungus.

The box of **baking soda** you keep in the fridge to absorb odors can relieve the itch and burn between your toes or on your feet. Add enough water to one tablespoon of baking soda to make a paste. Rub in the paste, then rinse and thoroughly dry your feet. Finish up with a dusting of **cornstarch** or **powder**.

For a soothing foot soak, add two teaspoons of **salt** to one pint of warm water. Soak your feet for 5 to 10 minutes. Repeat this soak at frequent intervals until your feet are completely healed.

Tea contains tannic acid, a natural astringent that works wonderfully to dry out sweaty feet. Steep five tea bags in a quart of boiling water for five minutes. Let cool to lukewarm, then soak your feet in this "tea bath" for 30 minutes.

A soothing compress containing a mild astringent can ease itching and burning and help dry up blisters. Mix one packet of **Domeboro powder** or two tablespoons **Burow's solution** (both contain aluminum acetate and are available in drugstores) into one pint of cold water. Soak a white cotton cloth in the solution and apply it three or four times a day for 15 to 20 minutes at a time.

Don't Give Fungus a New Home

The tinea fungus that causes athlete's foot is also the cause of notorious jock itch. That's why, when you have athlete's foot, you need to be careful not to infect your groin area. Make certain you thoroughly clean your hands after touching your feet. And don't pull your undies on over your bare feet. Put on your socks first. If you wear pantyhose, put on socks, don your drawers, remove the socks, and put on the hose.

Fight Fungus with Food

Plain **yogurt** containing live acidophilus bacteria is an instant remedy for athlete's foot. These friendly microorganisms keep the fungus in check. Simply dab the yogurt on the infected areas, let dry, and rinse off. (But don't use the flavored kind!)

Add a few drops of **mustard** oil or a bit of mustard powder to a footbath. Mustard will help to kill the fungus. Soak your feet in the bath for up to half an hour.

Seek Herbal Relief

The oil of the Australian tea tree is a potent antiseptic. It alters the environment of the skin, making it harder for tinea to do its nasty work. For a soothing, healing treatment, mix **tea-tree oil** with the same amount of **olive oil** and rub the combination into the affected area twice a day. The olive oil helps to tenderize skin toughened by athlete's foot so the tea-tree oil is better absorbed.

Alternatively, mix **tea-tree oil** with **aloe gel**, another skin softener. Mix three parts tea-tree oil to one part aloe gel and rub this salve into the infected area twice a day. Give this treatment six to eight weeks to work.

The heavenly scented herb **lavender** also has anti-fungal properties. Make a massage oil by adding three drops of lavender oil to one teaspoon of carrier oil (any vegetable oil or skin lotion will do). Rub into the infected skin daily.

Calendula has been valued for centuries as a topical treatment for wounds and skin conditions. This herbal healer is said to have both antifungal and anti-inflammatory powers. Rub calendula ointment, sold at health-food stores, on the affected areas, especially between your toes.

Should I call **the doctor?**

Give home treatments at least three weeks to work. If your symptoms are severe, however, get to a dermatologist or podiatrist. Left untreated, a fungal infection can cause the skin to crack, which allows infection-causing bacteria to gain entry. You should also get to the doctor as soon as possible if you see signs of a more serious infection such as skin that is angry red and tender to the touch or oozing. Other warning signals are swelling of the foot or leg accompanied by a fever, or red streaks radiating from the infected area.

Tried...

Some people claim that they've used their own saliva to cure athlete's foot.

...and true

Studies in animals suggest that saliva does appear to have antibacterial and antifungal powers. For example, when the salivary glands of rats are removed, their wounds heal more slowly, and a dog's saliva kills bacteria that can cause infections in newborn puppies. Human saliva contains substances called histatins, shown to have antifungal activity.

The Power of Prevention

⤻ After a bath or shower, **dry your feet thoroughly.** You might try using a blow-dryer, particularly between your toes.

⤻ Wear clean white socks made of natural fiber—they absorb moisture best—or synthetics designed to **draw moisture away from the foot.** If you can, change your socks during the day to keep your feet sweat-free.

⤻ Wear shoes made of canvas or leather, which **allow your feet to breathe.** Forgo rubber and plastic, which hold moisture in and can cause feet to sweat.

⤻ Don't wear the same shoes two days in a row. It takes at least a day for shoes to dry out. If your feet sweat heavily, **change your shoes** twice a day.

⤻ Dust the insides of your shoes with **antifungal powder** or spray. To kill fungus spores, spray some **disinfectant,** like Lysol, on a cloth and wipe out the insides of your shoes after you take them off.

⤻ **Wear slippers** or **shower shoes** in places where others go barefoot, like gyms, health clubs, locker rooms, and around swimming pools.

⤻ If your toenails are thick, yellow, crumbly, and brittle, you may have a fungal nail infection, which can lead to athlete's foot. **Kick the toenail fungus**—with either an over-the-counter antifungal medication or a visit to your podiatrist or dermatologist—and you'll reduce your chances of getting athlete's foot.

Back Pain

"Oh, my aching back!" Wish you never had to utter those words again? Take it easy for a couple of days while taking some ibuprofen or naproxen sodium to ease swelling and relieve the pain. Also try the fast-acting solutions below—especially ice and heat—for immediate relief. Then, as soon as possible, slowly get moving again. When your back is feeling moderately better, do some gentle stretching and strengthening exercises and in four to six weeks your back should be back in action.

Ice First, Heat Later

⟿ As a pain reliever, **ice** works great. It temporarily blocks pain signals and helps reduce swelling. Several times a day, lay an ice pack wrapped in a towel on the painful area for up to 20 minutes. Alternatively, you can use a bag of **frozen peas** or **corn**. During the first few days of home treatment, apply the ice pack as frequently as necessary. Later you may still want to use ice after exercise or physical activities.

⟿ After about 48 hours, switch to **moist heat** to stimulate blood flow and reduce painful spasms. Dip a towel in very warm water, wring it out, then flatten and fold it. Lie on your stomach with pillows under your hips and ankles. Place the towel across the painful area, cover the towel with plastic wrap, then put a heating pad—set on medium—atop the plastic. Leave it on for up to 20 minutes. You can repeat this three or four times a day for several days.

Rub In Some Relief

⟿ Ask a partner to **massage** the aching area. If you want to use a "back rub" cream or ointment, go ahead, but use caution, as most topical creams produce skin irritation after a few applications. For a simple back-massage aid, stuff several tennis balls into a long sock, tie the end of the sock, and have your partner roll it over your back.

What's wrong

Something's amiss with the delicate column of bones, muscles, ligaments, and joints that holds you up. You might have strained a muscle, pulled a ligament, or maybe you have a herniated disk. These disks, which separate the vertebrae, are fibrous rings surrounding a pulpy core. If a disk is herniated, some of that pulpy material is pushing against a nerve root. You have sciatica if a herniated disk presses on the sciatic nerve, causing sharp pain to shoot down the leg. But there are numerous other causes of back pain: strains, arthritis, hairline spine fractures, even kidney infections.

Before you try any home remedies or exercises, see a doctor to find out whether you have a common type of lower back pain or a medical problem that requires special treatment. A good physical therapist or chiropractor can help stop the back spasm by applying traction and gentle manipulation. Also call the doctor if pain comes on suddenly, radiates down your leg to your knee or foot, or if it's accompanied by fever, stomach cramps, chest pain, or labored breathing. Doctors consider back pain a wake-up call, and will usually recommend a spine stabilization and strengthening program to help prevent future problems.

Rub on creams containing **methyl salicylate.** Derived from the wintergreen shrub, it's a natural pain reliever related to aspirin. Often combined with menthol or camphor, it's a common ingredient in many liniments such as Ben-Gay, ArthriCare, Heet Liniment, and Icy Hot cream. The creams, called counterirritants, stimulate nerve endings in the skin, distracting you from deeper pain. When you use them, you're also giving yourself a massage—and that hands-on pressure combined with the surface action packs a one-two punch. (*Off-limits* . . . if you're also using heating pads or hot compresses on the area.)

Pick a pepper product. Your drugstore carries creams such as Capsin, Pain-X, ThermoRub Lotion, and Zostrix that contain **capsaicin,** the heat-producing substance in hot peppers. Applied to your skin, capsaicin depletes nerve endings of a neurochemical called substance P. Researchers have found that substance P is essential for transmitting pain sensations to the brain, so when there's less substance P in circulation, the pain meter is turned down a bit. Look for a cream or ointment containing 0.075% or 0.025% capsaicin. And be patient: You may have to use it for several weeks to feel the full effect. Stop using it if you begin to feel any skin irritation.

Swallow These Soothers

Three or four times a day, take 500 milligrams of **bromelain.** Derived from pineapples, this enzyme promotes circulation, reduces swelling, and helps your body reabsorb the by-products of inflammation. Look for a strength between 1,200 and 2,400 MCU (milk-clotting units) or 720 and 1,440 GDU (gelatin-dissolving units). Wait for at least an hour after each meal before taking the bromelain, or it will work mainly in your gut instead of your muscles.

Try taking one 250-milligram capsule of **valerian** four times a day. Some scientists claim that this herb's active ingredient interacts with receptors in the brain to cause a sedating effect. Although sedatives are not generally recommended, valerian is much milder than any pharmaceutical product. (Valerian can also be made into a tea, but the smell is so strong—resembling overused gym socks—that capsules are vastly preferable.)

Fast Relief from the Doc

Doctors used to prescribe muscle relaxers for quick relief, but the drugs are rarely prescribed anymore. They tend to make people tired and contribute to poor muscle tone and coordination—just the opposite of what you really need for back-pain relief.

If you visit your doctor or hospital to be treated for intense pain, you're more likely to be given a drug called Toradol. This powerful, prescription anti-inflammatory and pain reliever stops the muscle spasms and relieves pain.

Perfect Your Posture

➤ Look for the **posture that places the least stress** on your back. To do it, stand straight with your weight evenly balanced on both feet. Tilt your pelvis forward, then back, exaggerating the movement. Then settle into the position that feels most comfortable. Now "work your way up" your back, focusing on one area at a time. First concentrate on the area near your waist, then your chest area, and finally your neck and shoulders. Try to feel which position is least stressful and most comfortable. This is the position to maintain when you're standing, walking, and beginning or ending any exercise.

➤ **When you're sleeping**, lie on your back or your side (*unless* you have sciatica). If you're more comfortable on your back, place a pillow under your knees as well as under your head to relieve pressure on your lower back. Prefer to sleep on your side? Place a pillow between your legs. For anyone who has sciatica, the recommended sleeping position is on your stomach.

➤ If you like to sit up in bed to read or watch TV, get a **large foam wedge** that couches your upper body in a comfortable position. For added comfort—and to keep your neck in the proper position—use a foam or inflatable neck support when you're sitting up.

➤ When you're seated in a chair at the office or home, keep your feet flat on the floor, with your hips slightly higher than your knees. Use a **lumbar support** behind your lower back. The lumbar roll is a chair-width foam cylinder about five inches in diameter. You can improvise with a rolled-up towel, but the foam product is lighter, easier to position, and usually has straps that attach to the back of the chair.

Tried...

In frontier days, a mustard plaster was a favorite remedy for sore backs and aching joints.

...and true

Like capsaicin and other counter-irritants, mustard delivers a warm, tingling sensation that can distract you from deeper pain. To make a plaster, mix one part powdered mustard with two parts flour, adding water until you have a paste. Spread it on a dishcloth, then fold the cloth and apply it like a compress to your skin. It can burn if left on too long, so remove it if you feel skin discomfort. Don't use a mustard plaster more than three times a day.

Sciatica: What's the Connection?

The roots of the sciatic nerve lie near the base of your spine. They pass through a tunnel in your pelvis called the sciatic notch, then come together like separate lanes merging into superhighways—the two large sciatic nerves that lead all the way down your legs. When the sciatic roots are pinched—by pressure from a herniated disk, for instance—sensations of pain, tingling, or numbness may extend all the way from your buttocks to your legs, feet, and toes.

About half the people who have sciatica get good results from most of the treatments recommended for lower back pain. If you have sciatica and don't get relief with these treatments, however, you should keep your doctor informed. And tell your doctor at once if you start to have trouble controlling your bladder or bowels. In a small percentage of cases (5 to 10 percent), doctors may recommend other procedures, such as surgery.

➤ Keep a **foam wedge** in the car and place it behind your lower back whenever you're seated.

➤ If you're accustomed to walking around with **a wallet** in your hip pocket, **take it out** whenever you're sitting. Even though it feels like a small lump, it's big enough to tilt your backside, throwing your spine ever so slightly out of alignment.

➤ When you're standing at the sink doing dishes, or waiting in a long line, **raise one foot higher than the other.** In the kitchen, keep a low sturdy box or a couple of old books by the sink, and put up a foot while you're standing there. Waiting in line, use a step or curb. (Think of the traditional brass rail in a bar, which serves the same purpose.) Periodically change position by putting up the opposite foot. This shifting of weight gives alternating back muscles a chance to relax.

Rise and Shine

➤ Each morning before **you get out of bed**, lie on your back and slowly stretch your arms overhead. Gently pull your knees to your chest, one at a time. To rise, roll to the edge of your bed, turn on your side, put your knees over the edge, and use one arm to push yourself up as you let your feet swing to the floor. Once you're on your feet, put your hands on your buttocks and lean back very slowly to stretch out your spine.

Bad Breath

Suppose you conduct a "breath test" as you head to an important encounter, and you flunk. Don't worry—the following fast fixes can help tame your wild-and-woolly breath. If odor-causing bacteria seem to be fond of your gums, tongue, and teeth, you'll want to adopt some daily habits to inhibit these inhabitants. That's when special rinses, attention to toothpaste, and faithful brushing and flossing can begin making bad breath good.

Take Emergency Measures

꙰ Dry mouth is a haven for the bacteria that cause bad breath. So find a tap, and swish the **water** around in your mouth. Water will temporarily dislodge bacteria and make your breath a bit more palatable.

꙰ At the end of your power lunch or romantic dinner, munch the sprig of **parsley** that's left on your plate. Parsley is rich in chlorophyll, a known breath deodorizer with germ-fighting qualities.

꙰ If you can get your hands on an **orange**, peel and eat it. The citric acid it contains will stimulate your salivary glands and encourage the flow of breath-freshening saliva.

꙰ If there are no oranges in sight, **eat whatever is available**, except known breath-foulers like garlic, onions, or a stinky cheese. Eating encourages the flow of saliva, which helps remove the unpleasant, odor-causing material on the back of your tongue.

꙰ Vigorously **scrape your tongue** over your teeth. Your tongue can become coated with bacteria that ferment proteins, producing gases that smell bad. Scraping your tongue can dislodge these bacteria so you can rinse them away.

꙰ If you have a metal or plastic spoon, use it as a **tongue scraper.** To scrape safely, place the spoon on the back of your tongue and drag it forward. Repeat four or five times. Scrape the sides of the tongue as well, with the same back-to-front

What's **wrong**

People are backing away from you whenever you stop to talk with them. Or someone has told you frankly that you have bad breath. The most obvious cause: You've eaten a dish laced with onions, garlic, or blue cheese. But there are other reasons galore. Perhaps you're a smoker or could it be that you don't brush your teeth or floss often enough? Gum disease is another common cause of bad breath. If you have an abscessed tooth or a sinus infection, your unpleasant breath is most certainly a side effect. Rounding out the list of suspects: certain medications, a chronically dry mouth, or too many cups of coffee.

Should I call
the doctor?

While all of us have mal-odorous breath from time to time, good oral hygiene should keep it to a minimum. But bad breath that hangs on can also be a sign of intestinal problems, cancer, or lung or kidney problems. If you brush and floss diligently, yet can't banish bad breath on your own, place a call to your doctor or dentist. And see a doctor if your breath smells sweet or fruity, since that's one sign of diabetes.

motion. Don't push the spoon too far back, however; you may activate your gag reflex.

Raid the Spice Shelf

🌿 **Cloves** are rich in eugenol, a potent antibacterial. Simply pop one into your mouth and dent it with your teeth. The pungent aromatic oil may burn slightly, so keep that spicy nub moving. Continue to bite until the essence permeates your mouth, then spit it out. Don't use clove oil or powdered cloves; they're too strong and can cause burns.

🌿 Chew on **fennel, dill, cardamom,** or **anise seeds.** Anise, which tastes like black licorice, can kill the bacteria that grow on the tongue. The others can help mask the odor of halitosis.

🌿 Suck on a stick of **cinnamon.** Like cloves, cinnamon is effective as an antiseptic.

Choose Your Fresheners

🌿 The most obvious brand-name products advertised as breath-fresheners are rarely, if ever, effective in the long run. But with a **chlorine dioxide** rinse, you can dismantle the sulfur compounds that are responsible for breath odor. These products are available both at your local drugstore and over the Internet. One brand, TheraBreath, is available at pharmacies. Another, ProFresh, can be purchased at www.profresh.com.

🌿 Use a toothpaste that contains **tea-tree oil,** a natural disinfectant. If you can't find it in the pharmacy, look for it in health-food stores.

The Power of Prevention

🌿 Use an **oral irrigator,** which is a handheld device that rapidly pulses a small jet of water into your mouth, to flush out

How to Sniff Out Bad Breath

Just how bad is your breath? To find out, cup your hands over your mouth, exhale heartily, and take a whiff. If your breath smells bad to you, it smells bad to others too. You can also perform the "sniff test" on dental floss after you pull it gently between your teeth. But if you think you might have become desensitized to your own bad breath, you can ask your dentist to test you with a halimeter. This device measures the sulfur content of your breath—which is what makes it smell bad.

the bad bacteria, which can go deeper than a brush or floss string can reach.

➤ Carry a **toothbrush** with you and brush immediately after every meal. With prompt brushing you thwart the development of plaque, the soft, sticky film that coats the teeth and gums.

➤ To keep your toothbrush free of stink-triggering bacteria, store it, head down, in a lidded plastic tumbler of **hydrogen peroxide.** Rinse the brush well before you use it.

➤ If you wear **dentures,** it's possible that they are absorbing the bad odors in your mouth. Always soak them overnight in an **antiseptic solution,** unless your dentist has advised you otherwise.

➤ **Don't skip meals.** When you don't eat for a long period of time, your mouth can get very dry. It becomes a perfect breeding ground for bacteria.

➤ Some things can sour your breath even if there are no bacteria in the neighborhood. These include cigarettes, alcohol, onions, garlic, and especially strong cheeses like Camembert, Roquefort, and blue cheese. In situations where sweet breath is a must, use the commonsense approach—just say no.

➤ Ask your doctor if a **medication** could be fouling the air you expel. Any drug that dries out your mouth, thereby depriving it of saliva, is suspect. These include over-the-counter antihistamines, decongestants, diet pills, and prescription medications for depression and high blood pressure.

Skip it!

It's a common misconception that minty mouthwash or breath mints will turn your breath fresh. Not so. Most mouthwashes contain alcohol, which dries up saliva. When you use them, you actually make your breath worse afterward. And mint candy is just a cover-up; it actually feeds the odor-causing bacteria more sugar! For a natural mouthwash that won't dry out your mouth, mix 1 tablespoon baking soda with 1 cup of a 2%–3% solution of hydrogen peroxide. The foam it kicks up has a powerful oxidizing effect that kills odoriferous bacteria.

Blisters

The eternal dilemma: Should I drain this thing or leave it alone? In general, don't bother blisters that are small or those that probably won't pop on their own. They are less likely to become infected if you leave the natural covering intact, and under the sheltering cushion of fluid, the area has time to form new skin. Meanwhile, follow these tips to relieve the pain and itching and speed healing. If your blister is large, or in a spot where you can't avoid putting pressure on it, drain it the proper way. Never pop a burn blister, though. There's a serious risk of infection if you do.

What's wrong

You've most likely rubbed your skin the wrong way...literally. The most frequent cause of blisters is excessive friction on moist skin. As a blister forms, clear fluid accumulates in a pocket between the layers of the skin. Sometimes a small blood vessel in the area is damaged, and the fluid in the blister becomes tinged with blood. These types of blisters are generally found on the hands and feet, but can occur elsewhere too. Other potential blister causes include poison ivy and oak, sunburn and other burns, and eczema and other skin conditions.

Let It Be

⌁ Keep the blister clean with soap and water. You can dab on **petroleum jelly** or some other emollient to minimize further friction.

⌁ Cover the blister with a clean **bandage** that you change at least once a day.

⌁ Protect the blister with a piece of **moleskin**—a soft, adhesive cushion that's sold in pharmacies. (Don't worry—no real moles have been sacrificed to make this product.) Leave it on for two days, and remove it carefully so it doesn't tear the fragile skin beneath.

⌁ Apply **calendula ointment**, a product made from marigold. It's traditionally used as a soothing wound healer. To keep the ointment clean, cover it with an adhesive bandage or a gauze pad. At night, remove the bandage so the blistered area is exposed to air.

⌁ No calendula? Smear some **aloe vera gel** on the blister and cover it with a bandage to help it heal. But be sure you use the pure gel of the plant. Some processed products contain ingredients, like alcohol, which have a drying effect.

⌁ Another option for blister treatment is **Preparation H.** While this isn't the normal use for the hemorrhoid reliever, the cream has ingredients that relieve itching and burning, and it provides a coating that protects the skin.

🍂 Relieve pain and itching with a **wet washcloth.** Soak the cloth in cold water, wring it out, and lay it over the blister.

If It Pops by Accident...

🍂 Wash it with soap and water. Apply a healing cream or gel like **Neosporin** or **Betadine.** Cover it with a bandage. Four times a day, remove the bandage and treat the raw spot with a mixture of one part **tea-tree oil** and three parts **vegetable oil.** The tea-tree oil will help kill bacteria and prevent an infection.

Practice the Art of Careful Draining

🍂 If your blister is large, or in a spot where you can't avoid putting pressure on it, you may be better off **draining** it rather than trying to protect it. To drain a blister properly, first sterilize a needle. Use a pair of pliers or tweezers to hold the needle over a flame for a few seconds until it glows red. Let it cool.

🍂 Clean the blister with **rubbing alcohol** or a disinfecting product like **Betadine.**

🍂 Open a **sterile gauze pad** and lay it gently on top of the blister. Pierce the edge of the blister, sliding the needle in sideways, and gently squeeze out the liquid by pressing down on the gauze pad. Make sure you don't tear or remove that top layer of skin—it's protecting an extremely sensitive circle of skin beneath.

🍂 Smear on an antibiotic ointment like **Neosporin** and cover it with a clean bandage. You can also cover it with a **2nd Skin Moist Burn Pad**, made by Spenco. This is a moist, jelly-like covering that can be cut to size and taped in place. Change it twice a day.

🍂 If the blister refills again later, **drain it again** the same way.

🍂 Apply a mixture of **vitamin E** and **calendula ointment** to help your skin heal faster. Vitamin E comes in gel capsules. Slice open a capsule, mix equal amounts of the vitamin and calendula oil, and smear the mixture on your blister. Reapply as needed for up to a week.

The Power of Prevention

🍂 Don't assume you know your proper shoe size or that your feet haven't changed since you last bought shoes. **Have**

Should I call **the doctor?**

If your blister is extremely large—more than two inches across—you should seek medical care. Symptoms of infection should also send you to the doctor. These include prolonged pain that isn't fading, fever, redness that extends beyond the borders of the blister, yellow crusting, and oozing pus. Some disorders that cause blisters, such as chicken pox, eczema, and impetigo, also may require a doctor's care.

Felled by a Blister

your feet measured every time you buy. And when you try on shoes, be sure you're wearing the same kind of socks you normally wear.

⏱ Shop for shoes in the **afternoon.** Your feet swell during the day, and if you buy a pair in the morning, you might be getting a half-size too small.

⏱ Be sure new shoes are **roomy in the toe area.** When you're standing up, you should have a thumb-width of space between your longest toe and the end of your shoe.

⏱ For long walks or hikes, try wearing **two pairs of socks** to reduce friction. The inner pair should be a thin, sweat-wicking fabric like acrylic, with an outer sock made of cotton.

⏱ You may also want to **use an antiperspirant** on your feet to keep them dry. Dry feet are less likely to develop blisters.

⏱ Cover blister-prone spots with a lubricant, such as **Lube-Stick for Runners,** before you go for a run.

⏱ If you're going to be doing yard work, you can prevent blisters on your hands by wearing **work gloves.** If you always get blisters when you weed the garden, even if you wear gloves, shop for a weeder with a larger handle or a cushioned grip.

⏱ Anyone who plays racket sports will probably have to contend with hand blisters. But if they keep recurring, talk to a pro about **changing the grip** on your racket or wrapping it with an absorbent, soft covering.

Body Odor

All's swell that ends smell. If antiperspirants (which plug up sweat glands) and deodorants (which mask odors) don't do the trick, or you prefer a natural approach, there are myriad paths to an agreeable essence. BO battles begin in the shower and continue throughout the day, with a simple goal: Stop the odor at its source.

Watch the Daily Soaps

↪ Pick an **antibacterial soap**, such as Dial, Lifebuoy, or Lever 2000. These leave ingredients on your skin that kill bacteria even after you're finished bathing. If the soap doesn't irritate your skin, use it daily. If you find that these soaps are too drying, use them only on your underarms and groin, where you need their antibacterial power the most.

↪ If BO is still bothering you, bring out the big guns. **Betadine**, an antibacterial cleanser, is so effective that some formulations are used to clean patients before surgery. Since it can dry your skin, however, you should use it in the shower, where it will rinse off quickly, and only on high-smell areas such as the armpits and groin. Squeeze out a small amount of cleanser, wash the target areas first, then rinse off the Betadine and finish your shower with regular soap.

↪ Another, milder antibacterial formulation is **Hibiclens**. It's gentler on the skin than Betadine.

Beyond Deodorant

↪ Wipe **rubbing alcohol, vinegar,** or **hydrogen peroxide** onto your underarms during the day to cut down the numbers of odor-causing bacteria.

↪ Dab on **witch hazel.** You can splash it directly on your skin or apply it as often as necessary with a cotton pad. The clear, clean-smelling liquid has drying and deodorizing properties.

↪ Dust **baking soda** or **cornstarch** on any odor-troubled part of your body. Both of these powders absorb moisture, and baking soda also kills odor-causing bacteria.

What's **wrong**?

Long ago, nature provided us with strong smells to entice the opposite sex. But BO won't get you far today. The problem starts with certain types of sweat. *Eccrine glands* pour out clear, neutral-smelling sweat, which cools your body as it evaporates. *Apocrine glands,* concentrated in your underarms and genitals, secrete a substance that bacteria feast upon, causing strong odors. Stress, ovulation, sexual excitement, and anger can cause apocrine glands to kick into high gear. Some diseases cause the body to produce particular odors, and so do drugs such as venlafaxine (Effexor) and bupropion (Wellbutrin).

Should I call
the doctor?

If you're sweating frequently or heavily, you could have an overactive thyroid gland, low blood sugar, or a problem with the part of the nervous system that controls sweating. If you think you're sweating too much or you may have a medical condition causing your body odor, see your doctor. And if you're taking a prescription medication that might be contributing to excessive odor, ask your doctor about switching to another drug.

Did you
know?

Hunters often use special soaps to mask all traces of human odor so their keen-smelling quarry won't smell them. You can try this approach so *human* noses won't notice you. Look for the products in hunting stores or catalogs.

⤙ **Shave regularly** under your arms. Underarm hair can increase body odor because it traps sweat and bacteria.

Help from the Garden

⤙ Apply **tea-tree oil** to problem areas, as long as it doesn't irritate your skin. This oil, from an Australian tree, kills bacteria and also has a pleasant scent.

⤙ Essential oils of **lavender, pine,** and **peppermint** fight bacteria. They also smell nice. Since some people have a skin reaction to certain oils, test the underarm area or a small patch of skin before using.

⤙ Delightfully fragrant, **sage** can fight bacteria and reduce perspiration. You can purchase a solution of sage tincture or diluted sage oil, or brew some sage tea that you cool and store in a bottle. Any of these liquids can be used in the underarm area, but not around the genitals. And after using sage, wash your hands before touching your face.

⤙ A citrus fruit like **lemon** changes the pH level of your skin, making it more acidic. All bacteria, including the odor-causing kinds, have a hard time surviving in a highly acidic environment. Just rub on some lemon and pat dry.

Eat Green, Smell Clean

⤙ Eat plenty of **spinach, chard,** and **kale.** Green, leafy vegetables are rich in chlorophyll, which has a powerful deodorizing effect in your body.

⤙ Have a few sprigs of **parsley,** credited with anti-odor properties. Or make parsley tea by steeping a teaspoon of chopped fresh parsley in a cup of boiling water for five minutes. Let it cool a bit before you drink it.

⤙ Try **wheatgrass juice,** sold in health-food stores. Warning: It has a very strong taste, and some people feel nauseated the first time they try it. You might want to start with just an ounce of wheatgrass juice in six ounces of water, then increase the proportion of juice in subsequent tastings. On first tasting, it's wise to try this drink on an empty stomach just in case your stomach overreacts.

⤙ Buy tablets containing **chlorophyll.** Many brands are available, made from plants like kelp, barley grass, and blue-green algae. Check the label for the dosage recommendation.

Bronchitis

Your goal: Thin the phlegm in your chest and get it moving, so you can cough it up and out. The most direct approach to your lungs is the air you breathe, so inhalation treatments are a first resort. Think of them as a steam cleaning for your airways. The right food and drink can also help to keep mucus on the move. At the same time, you'll want to get some germ-fighters into your body's ecosystem so the bugs that cling to that mucus are mightily discouraged. Here's how to proceed:

Have Good Self-Steam

➤ **Breathe steam.** You can do that just by taking a hot shower, of course. Or pour steaming-hot water into a bowl and lean over it, draping a towel over your head. Inhaling the steam will help loosen the secretions in your lungs.

➤ To make the steam treatment even more effective, add a few drops of **eucalyptus** or **pine oil** to the water. Eucalyptus helps to soften mucus in obstructed airways and has some antibacterial properties. (If you want to use eucalyptus leaves, simply boil them in a pot of water, then remove from the heat and inhale the steam.) Pine oil acts as an expectorant, so it will help you "bring up" phlegm from the bronchial tubes.

➤ Run a **humidifier** in your bedroom when you're sleeping to moisten the air you breathe. But be sure to follow the manufacturer's directions for cleaning the humidifier. Otherwise, bacteria and mold can accumulate in the works.

➤ If you have an ultrasound, cool-mist humidifier, add the contents of a one-pint bottle of **3% hydrogen peroxide** and a quarter-cup of water. The hydrogen peroxide works to thin mucus and may even help get the infection under control. You can leave the humidifier running day and night so you're constantly breathing in the vapors.

Make a Run for It

➤ To thin mucus and help you cough it up more easily, **drink lots of water**—at least eight 8-ounce glasses each day.

What's wrong

Short-lived cases of bronchitis are usually caused by a viral or bacterial infection, though they can also be brought on by allergies. The bronchial tubes swell up, and the cilia—tiny hairs lining the respiratory tract—become paralyzed. Mucus accumulates, forcing you to cough heavily. You may also experience achiness, shortness of breath, wheezing, sweating, chills, fatigue, and fever. These symptoms generally go away after 10 days. Chronic bronchitis, on the other hand, can last a lifetime. Most chronic bronchitis is caused by cigarette smoking, though some cases originate from exposure to fumes and dust.

Should I call
the doctor?

See your doctor if your
cough is interfering
with your sleep or your
normal routine, or if
breathing is difficult.
You should also call the
doctor if you have a fever
above 100 degrees or
you're coughing up blood.
Bronchitis can lead to
pneumonia.

And **avoid alcohol** and caffeinated drinks, which dehydrate your system and make the mucus tougher to dislodge.

 Eat **chile peppers, hot spicy salsa,** or dishes prepared with **cayenne pepper.** Fiery foods don't just make your nose run—they also thin the mucus in your lungs, helping you cough more productively.

 Drink **mullein tea.** Mullein, a traditional folk remedy for respiratory ailments, offers another way to clear mucus from your lungs. It contains saponins, which help loosen phlegm, along with a gelatinous mucilage that soothes raw mucous membranes. Boil a cup of water, remove from the heat, and drop in two teaspoons dried mullein leaves. Let the tea steep for 10 minutes, then strain out the wet leaves and drink the tea. You can drink up to three cups a day.

 Avoid milk products. Cow's milk contains lactalbumin, which stimulates the production of mucus in the upper and lower respiratory tract and in the intestines. (Young calves, with four stomachs, need this extra mucus to help protect their intestinal tracts from strong stomach acids . . . but you don't!) When humans drink cow's milk, the result is excessive mucus production.

Supplement Your Efforts

 N-acetyl cysteine (NAC), a form of the amino acid cysteine, helps thin and loosen mucus. Take one 600-milligram dose three times daily, between meals, until the bronchitis has cleared up. If you're treating short-lived bronchitis, continue taking NAC for another few weeks after the cough goes away.

 Echinacea and **astragalus** are herbs that strengthen the immune system and help you fight off bacteria and viruses. Take 500 milligrams of either herb four times a day for acute bronchitis or twice daily for chronic bronchitis.

 R-lipoic acid is a powerful antioxidant nutrient that is vital in the repair of inflamed airways. Like other antioxidants such as vitamins E and C, R-lipoic acid contributes to your health by counteracting the effects of harmful molecules called free radicals, which damage cells. Usually your body produces enough lipoic acid on its own, but when there's inflammation, cells are under stress and need all the help they can get. Take 100 milligrams of R-lipoic acid three times daily with meals.

A medicinal formula called **Arcozon** has potent antibacterial and immune-stimulating properties. It contains four herbs that have been traditionally used by healers in the Amazon rainforest: *uña de gato* (cat's claw), pau d'arco, suma, and jatoba. You can use it to prevent or treat bronchial infections. Take one teaspoon or four capsules four times daily for short-lived bronchitis or twice daily for chronic bronchitis.

The Power of Prevention

To prevent chronic bronchitis, the most essential advice is: **Don't smoke.** If you're a smoker, find out about programs that will help you give it up.

If your job exposes you to lots of dust, fumes, or pollutants—any of which can contribute to chronic bronchitis—be sure you're wearing the proper **mask** or **respirator** to filter the impurities from the air you breathe.

To slash your risk of getting viral bronchitis, **wash your hands** frequently and keep them away from your face, especially when you've been around someone who has a cold.

Clean your nose and sinuses with saline nasal spray. Or use a sinus-clearing product like Aller-CLEAR, which helps prevent allergens and infectious agents from getting into your lungs.

Vitamin C helps you fight off respiratory viruses. It works well in conjunction with supplemental flavonoids, also called bioflavonoids. As a preventive measure, take up to 2,000 milligrams daily of vitamin C with flavonoids in divided doses. (With higher doses of vitamin C, some people get diarrhea.)

Skip it!

When you're coughing, it might seem like the most obvious treatment is a cough suppressant. But if you have a wet, productive cough, you shouldn't try to suppress it. Instead, use an expectorant cough syrup that helps loosen mucus, so the coughing clears out your bronchial passages. To make sure you're getting an expectorant, look for products containing the ingredient guaifenesin.

Bruises

Bang! That's going to leave a bruise. Though bruises eventually go away on their own, you can take steps to reduce the pain and encourage faster fading. First, reduce blood flow to the area with ice and compression to minimize discoloration. Next, use heat to boost circulation and help clear away the pooled blood. At the same time, as long as the skin isn't broken, a number of herbal ointments and compresses can help erase the evidence of a klutzy moment that left its mark.

What's wrong

You've had a bump, blow, or knock to your body that was hard enough to damage small blood vessels under your skin. Blood leaks out of these blood vessels, called capillaries, and seeps into the surrounding tissue. For a while you see the traditional black-and-blue colors, which are the trademark of most bruises. As the pooled blood gradually breaks down, the colors take on a full palette of hues, from purple to green and yellow. Normally, bruises will fade away in 10 to 14 days without any treatment.

Speed the Paling Process

 Apply **ice** as soon as possible. If you cool the blood vessels around the bruised area, less blood will leak out into the surrounding tissue. Many flexible ice packs are available, specifically designed for injuries, and most rough-and-tumble athletes have the foresight to keep a couple of them in the freezer. If you're not so equipped, soak a cloth in ice-cold water and lay it over the bruise for 10 minutes. Or use a bag of **frozen vegetables** wrapped in a towel. Take it off after 10 minutes, and wait 20 minutes or so before you reapply the ice pack so you don't overchill the skin underneath.

 If you've bruised your arm or leg, immediately wrap an **elastic bandage** around the bruised part. By squeezing the tissues underneath, the bandage helps prevent blood vessels from leaking. The bruise won't be quite as severe.

 Reduce blood flow to the bruise to minimize discoloration. If you bruise your leg, for instance, and you can take a time-out, settle into a couch or lounge chair with your leg up on a pillow, above heart level. If it's your arm that's bruised, try to keep it propped up above heart level whenever you're sitting.

Have a Heat Exchange

 After cooling the bruise for 24 hours, start applying heat to bring more circulation to the area and help clear away the pooled blood. Use an **electric heating pad** for 20 minutes several times a day. Be sure to follow the instructions on the heating pad: To avoid burns, it should go on top of—not under—the bruised limb.

⬝ Alternatively, you can apply a **warm compress** either under or over the bruised area. A hot-water bottle will work. Or use a compress that can be heated in a microwave, such as **Thera-Temp Microwavable Moist Heat Pack**, available at medical supply stores and on Internet sites.

⬝ A warm compress of **comfrey** can also offer comfort. Comfrey contains compounds that reduce swelling and promote the rapid growth of new cells. Make a warm herbal solution by pouring a pint of boiling water over an ounce of dried comfrey leaves or two ounces of fresh leaves. Steep for 10 minutes, then strain. This is for an external use only—it's *not* for drinking. Soak a gauze pad or a washcloth in the solution and apply it to the bruise for an hour. (*Off-limits* . . . if the skin is broken or you have an open wound.)

⬝ **Vinegar** mixed with warm water will help the healing process. Vinegar increases blood flow near the skin's surface, so it may help dissipate the blood that has pooled in the bruise area. **Witch hazel** will also do the trick.

Here's the Rub

⬝ **Arnica** is an herb that has long been recommended for bruises. It contains a compound that reduces inflammation and swelling. Apply arnica ointment or gel to the bruise daily.

⬝ Take a handful of fresh **parsley** leaves, crush them, and spread them over the bruise. Wrap the area with an elastic bandage. Some experts claim that parsley decreases inflammation, reduces pain, and can make the bruise fade more quickly.

⬝ Gently rub **St. John's wort** oil into the bruise. Though St. John's wort is often taken as a capsule or tea for mild

Should I call **the doctor?**

If your bruises appear mysteriously—that is, in places that you haven't even injured—be sure to see your doctor. Sometimes bruises are the mark of serious conditions like hemophilia, leukemia, and aplastic anemia. Consult your doctor if you have a bruise at a joint and it leads to swelling, if a bruise doesn't fade after a week, if it's accompanied by severe pain or fever, or if you get a bruise on the side of your head over your ear (this area fractures easily).

The Do-It-Yourselfer's Flexible Ice Pack

If you tend to like bumptious sports—or you clobber your shins at regular intervals—it helps to have an ice pack handy. To prepare one in advance, fill a resealable plastic bag with two cups water and one-third cup rubbing alcohol. Zip it shut and stick it in the freezer. Overnight it forms a slushy ice that will conform to any body part that gets damaged in the course of daily activities. ·

Be Selective About Pain Relievers

Don't reach for the aspirin bottle when you've just gotten a bruise—it can make things worse. Aspirin thins the blood, which means it will more easily gather under the skin and make that bruise even more alarming. The same applies to ibuprofen (found in Advil) and naproxen (found in Aleve). If you think you're getting too many bruises and you're also taking aspirin regularly (to reduce your risk of heart attack, for example), talk to your doctor about the problem but don't stop taking the aspirin on your own. For pain relief when you have a bruise, use acetaminophen, the ingredient found in Tylenol.

depression, the oil has long been known as a wound healer. It's rich in tannins, astringents that help shrink tissue and control capillary bleeding. For the best effect, start this treatment soon after the bruise occurs, and repeat it three times a day.

 Look for **vitamin K cream** in the drugstore. Your body needs vitamin K to help with blood clotting. Rub it into the bruise twice a day to prevent further bleeding.

Swallow, Please

 Bromelain, an enzyme found in pineapples, actually "digests" proteins involved in causing inflammation and inducing pain. Take 250 to 500 milligrams of bromelain daily between meals until the bruise has faded.

 Use a **homeopathic version of arnica.** As soon as you get the bruise, start taking one dose every four hours. Take four doses the first day, then reduce your dosages to two or three pills daily as the bruise fades.

The Power of Prevention

 If you feel like you bruise too easily, you may be deficient in **vitamin C.** It strengthens capillary walls so they're less likely to leak blood and make a bruise. Get additional vitamin C by eating more peppers and citrus fruit, and take a multivitamin.

 Increase your intake of **flavonoids** by eating more **carrots, apricots, and citrus fruits.** These help vitamin C work better in the body. Grape-seed extract is also a rich supplier of flavonoids. Take 20 to 50 milligrams daily.

 People who are susceptible to bruising may be deficient in **vitamin K**, which you can get from broccoli, Brussels sprouts, and leafy green vegetables, as well as from supplements.

Bursitis and Tendinitis

There's nothing worse than having a much-valued limb go on strike, particularly if it's the one you rely on for gardening or golf, whittling or Wiffle Ball. The first lesson most athletes and weekend warriors need to learn is respect: Healing begins when you acknowledge the need for some time off from your usual activities. While you're on the mend, the name of the game is reducing the inflammation that's causing your soreness. Then you'll want to give your joint some TLC to ease it back into action and recover a full range of motion.

Make a Rest Stop

~ **Take a break** before you repeat the activity that triggered the pain. Be patient, since the problem may take a few weeks to resolve.

~ To hold down swelling, wrap an **elastic bandage** around the joint—but not too snugly. Then elevate the joint above the level of your heart. If it's your elbow that hurts, keep it on a high armrest, or sit in a low chair with your elbow propped up on the table. If you're treating your knee, lie on your back with the knee propped up on pillows.

Run Cold and Hot

~ **Ice your sore joint** to ease pain and inflammation. Wrap up an ice pack in a towel and apply it for 10 to 20 minutes every four hours. Or freeze a paper cup full of ice, tear off the top edge, and rub the ice where it hurts. Repeat three or four times a day, allowing two to five minutes for each treatment.

~ After about three days of giving joints the cold treatment—or until the joint is no longer warm to the touch—start **alternating cold with heat.** Heat increases blood flow to the injury, helping it to heal faster. Use a microwavable heat pack or an electric heating pad. Or, for form-fitting warmth, place two to three cups of rice in a large sock, tie off the sock, and microwave for 60 to 90 seconds. The rice will conform nicely to a knee, elbow, or ankle.

What's wrong

These somewhat related conditions are often the price you pay for too much repeated motion, whether something fun like playing tennis, or not so fun, like shoveling snow. Tendinitis is inflammation of the tendons, the tough cords that attach muscles to bones. Bursitis is inflammation of the bursae—tiny, fluid-filled sacs that provide cushioning where muscle touches bone or rubs up against another muscle. Where bursitis often feels like a dull ache at a joint, tendinitis tends to produce sharp pain. These conditions crop up most often in the shoulders, hips, elbows, knees, and ankles.

Should I call
the doctor?

If the problem gets worse after three or four days, or interferes with your daily activities, see your doctor. Also seek treatment if your joint is warm, red, and tender. These are signs of septic bursitis, a type of infection that can spread from one joint throughout your body.

Reach for Pain Relievers

∼ **Ibuprofen (Advil)** or **naproxen sodium (Aleve)** will help relieve the swelling and are very effective for short-term pain relief of this kind of pain.

∼ Try **boswellia.** Your body produces certain chemicals that actually increase pain. But this extract, from the frankincense tree, reduces your production of those chemicals. Take 400 to 500 milligrams three times a day. As your pain fades, cut down on the dosage.

∼ If you favor alternative approaches, consider a **homeopathic remedy.** If your joint is stiff and painful when you move it but feels better with more use, take a dose of **Rhus toxicodendron** at the 6C or 12C dilution every three to four hours until you feel relief. If the joint pain gets worse as you keep moving, take **bryonia** at the 6C or 12C dilution every three to four hours until the pain diminishes. For pain that comes on suddenly and acutely, homeopathic physicians recommend **ruta** and **arnica.** The recommended dose is a 6C or 12C dilution every three to four hours.

Take a Topical Vacation

∼ To soothe the aching area, rub on **arnica cream** or ointment—a remedy derived from the mountain daisy—two or three times a day. Also popular for treating bruises and sprains, arnica reduces swelling and inflammation. For even greater relief, press a hot-water bottle or heating pad against the joint after you've applied the arnica.

∼ **Tiger Balm**, a menthol-laced cream imported from China, can melt away pain. Rub it on the sore spot once or twice a day. But test a small patch of skin first. This is hot stuff, and some people develop a rash or redness if they use it too often.

∼ Use a soothing **ginger compress** to help stop the hurt from the outside in. Chop two tablespoons of fresh ginger, drop it in three cups of hot water, and let it steep for 20 minutes. Immerse a folded piece of cloth in the warm tea and wring it out. Lay the cloth over your sore joint for five minutes. Repeat three or four times a day.

🍃 **Vinegar**, applied topically, also eases aches. Soak a cloth or dishtowel in equal parts hot water and vinegar. Wring it out and apply.

Swallow Some Soothers

🍃 **Ginger** isn't just for compresses. Supplements of this natural anti-inflammatory can also help. For acute pain, take six 500-milligram capsules a day.

🍃 Give the "curry cure" a go. **Curcumin** is the active ingredient in turmeric, an Indian spice that's a key ingredient in curry. While turmeric has a venerable reputation as an anti-inflammatory and pain-relieving agent, it seems to be curcumin that does the real work—inhibiting the synthesis of prostaglandins, which are hormonelike compounds in the body involved in transmission of pain signals. Take 400 to 500 milligrams of the extract three times a day.

🍃 **Bromelain**, an enzyme from pineapple, reduces inflammation. The strength of the standardized extract is measured in milk-clotting units (MCU) or gelatin-dissolving units (GDU). Look for a product that contains between 1,200 and 2,400 MCU or between 720 and 1,440 GDU. Take 500 milligrams one hour after meals three or four times a day.

🍃 Consider **black cherry juice**, an old-time folk remedy. It contains an antioxidant plant pigment called quercetin, which works as an anti-inflammatory. Quaff 16 ounces a day, and there's a good chance your pain will dissipate.

🍃 Supplemental antioxidants will help strengthen and repair connective tissue in your joints. **Grape-seed** and **pine bark extract** are sources of powerful antioxidants called proanthocyanidins. Take 30 to 60 milligrams daily of both extracts.

🍃 **Manganese** helps the body clear away the waste products from inflammation related to bursitis or tendinitis. Take 50 to 100 milligrams of the mineral daily in divided doses for one or two weeks. If the pain continues, you can keep taking it for up to a month, but reduce the dose to 15 to 30 milligrams per day.

Favor the Fats That Coddle Your Joints

🍃 **Omega-3 fatty acids** help reduce inflammation. Increase the amounts in your diet by eating more cold-water fish, such as salmon, bluefin tuna, and mackerel. And consider taking supplemental flaxseed oil, which is rich in these "good" fats.

⌘ **Avoid** chips and other packaged foods that contain **hydrogenated oils**, and pass up fried foods, which are often cooked in those oils. These oils increase the inflammation in your body.

Ease into Sporting Life

⌘ As you resume sports or other normal activities, the joint that's been giving you pain will need some extra attention. Give the muscles near the joint a good **massage**—either on your own or with the help of a massage therapist—for additional pain relief and relaxation.

⌘ Always **stretch** properly before and after you exercise.

⌘ If you've had knee pain, make sure that you're using proper **shoes** for your sport. That's especially important before you resume a sport like tennis or running, where it's critical to have shoes that are well-fitting and in excellent condition. Get rid of those worn-out pairs that just have too many miles on them.

The Power of Prevention

⌘ Start a **strength-training** program using light weights to improve the muscles around the injured joint.

⌘ Avoid going to sleep with **your arm bent over your head**—that's a recipe for bursitis.

⌘ Be sure to interrupt long, repetitive chores with regular **stretch** breaks.

⌘ If you're a tennis player, avoid tennis elbow by making sure your racket has a large-handled grip and decreased string tension. Also, tennis elbow can develop if the racket head is too big or too small. Have the **grip, tension,** and **racket size** checked by a tennis instructor.

⌘ If you're going to be on your knees scrubbing the floor or pulling weeds, kneel on a **foam-rubber pad** designed for this purpose.

Calluses and Corns

In every pharmacy you'll find a section devoted to tender care of corns and calluses. This is a good aisle in which to start your search for relief. But the quest for treatment ingredients can take you much farther afield. If your feet are afflicted, you'll need the right oil to soften hard skin, customized patches for all-day protection, along with the socks, shoes, and insoles that protect you from pain. For hands, the right gloves count for a lot. Here's how to make corns and calluses take their lumps.

Wield a Stone and Board

➤ If a callus is causing you pain or aggravation, you need to scrape away some of those dead cells so the callus won't put so much pressure on your nerves. Immediately after a warm shower or bath, when your skin is wet and softened, rub a **pumice stone** on the callus to remove dead cells. A pumice stone, available at pharmacies, is simply a rough piece of volcanic mineral. Don't try to grind the whole callus away in one sitting, as you'll rub your skin raw. Instead, sand it down a little every day, and be patient. If the callus is very thick or hard, the sanding project might take a few weeks.

➤ For what are called "soft corns," use an **emery board.** Soft corns occur between your toes. They arise when the bones in adjacent toes rub until the skin thickens. A pumice stone won't fit in that tight space between toes. Instead, purchase the same kind of emery board that's designed to pare down fingernails and file away a little bit after every bath.

Soften Up the Opposition

➤ Instead of filing corns and calluses, you can soak and moisturize them until they grow soft. For corns on your toes, use **castor oil** as a softener with a **corn pad** as protector. To protect the corn, you want nonmedicated, doughnut-shaped pads, sold at pharmacies. Place one of these pads around the corn, dab a few drops of castor oil onto the corn with a cotton swab, then put adhesive tape over the top of the pad to hold it

What's **wrong**

When your body tries to defend itself from injury, it sometimes creates strange armor. The outermost layer of skin piles up a thick fortress of dead cells whenever it's rubbed too much or too often. That's what happens when an ill-fitting shoe keeps rubbing the same toe, or a metal-handled rake puts friction on the inside of your thumb. The epidermis gradually builds up a callus. That, in turn, can evolve into a corn, which is simply a callus with a hard core. Calluses on the hands and feet can be painless and protective. But if a callus or corn presses on a bone or nerve underneath your three layers of skin, it can be as painful as a pebble between your toes.

Should I call **the doctor?**

For anyone with diabetes, calluses and corns on the feet are particularly hazardous. Poor circulation puts you at high risk of foot infections, and it's dangerous to attempt self-treatment with nonsterile instruments that could introduce bacteria. So if you have diabetes, be sure to call your doctor whenever you have a callus or corn that needs attention. Others can probably try home treatments first, with the proviso that you need to get in touch with your doctor at once if the corn or callus becomes inflamed-looking. That's a sure sign of infection.

in place. The little padded doughnut encircles the corn and shields it from pressure while also holding in the moisturizing castor oil. (Since the castor oil can leak out through the bandage, causing stains, wear some old socks when you're using this treatment.)

~ Another good way to soften calluses and corns is to soak them in water containing **Epsom salt.** Follow the directions on the package.

Stalk the Corn with Acid

~ Look for medicated corn-removing patches that contain **salicylic acid.** Apply the patch after you've taken a shower. You might be able to leave on the patch until you shower again. But be sure to examine the area around the corn when you change the pad. The salicylic acid can cause sores on normal skin, and these can become infected.

~ Another source of salicylic acid is plain old **aspirin.** To create your own corn-softening compound, crush five aspirin until they turn into a fine powder. Mix the powder thoroughly with one-half teaspoon of lemon juice and one-half teaspoon water. Dab the paste onto the thickened skin, circle it with a piece of plastic wrap, then cover the plastic with a heated towel. Remove everything after 10 minutes and gently scrub away the loosened skin with a pumice stone.

Create Some Non-Friction

~ To help protect a callus or corn on your foot from pressure, custom-design a protective "doughnut" using a piece of adhesive **moleskin.** Cut a circle larger than your callus or corn, fold it in half, and cut a half-circle in the center. When you open it up, you'll have a padded ring. Apply it over your corn or callus.

~ If you have a soft corn between two toes, stick a **foam toe separator** between them to keep them from rubbing each other. Look for these in the foot-care section at the pharmacy.

~ Try socks that have very **thick, cushioned soles.** They could keep your calluses from getting worse.

~ Sometimes, adding an over-the-counter **insole** to your shoes—such as a Dr. Scholl's product—can decrease the pressure on the area with the callus, and help to resolve it more quickly.

The Power of Prevention

🌿 Apply a lotion containing **urea** to rough spots before they turn into troublesome calluses. **Carmol** is one brand. Start with a small amount, as urea-based lotions can sting.

🌿 Another way to prevent skin from toughening up is by soaking your feet in a tub of **warm water** once a week. Afterward, apply a **moisturizing lotion** such as Eucerin.

🌿 **Choose shoes that fit well.** You should have a thumb's width of distance between your longest toe and the end of the shoe. Shoes should be wide enough so that your toes and the balls of your feet aren't cramped from side to side. If shoes are too roomy, your feet slide around and rub against the sides.

🌿 Since feet naturally swell during the day, **shop for shoes late in the afternoon** when your feet are plumpest. If you shop in the early morning, you might get stuck with a pair of shoes that are too small.

🌿 For women, it's advisable to **save the high heels for special occasions.** Even for the grand soiree, however, you should choose high heels that have a lot of cushioning in the front to reduce pressure on your toes.

🌿 Don't play tennis in your running shoes. For each sport, select the **appropriate type of shoe.** A lot of research and engineering has gone into the development of shoes that are perfect for particular foot motions.

🌿 To prevent calluses on your hands, wear thickly cushioned **gloves** when you're doing work such as raking, painting, or pruning.

Skip it!

Some people may advise you to trim corns and calluses yourself, using a razor blade, scissors, or tweezers. Don't believe it! No matter how awesome your surgical skills, you have better things to do than practice on your own flesh. There's real danger of infection from mishandling sharp instruments.

Canker Sores

That little crater in your mouth causes more pain than anything so small deserves to. Rest assured that in a week or two, your canker sore will most likely be history, and you can chomp a chip, drink a cup of joe, or smooch your spouse without regretting it. Meanwhile, here are ways to blunt the pain and become a sore loser faster.

What's wrong

A mysterious condition known medically as recurrent aphthous stomatitis, canker sores typically appear inside the lips or cheeks, around the gums, or on the tongue. They are white or yellowish, with a halo of red, ranging from the size of a pinhead to the dimensions of a quarter. Experts aren't sure what causes them, but an immune-system malfunction is thought to play a role. A stressful episode or a mouth injury often precedes a breakout. Recurrent sores can also be brought on by eating certain foods.

Seal the Sore

 Over-the-counter products such as **Zilactin-B Canker Sore Gel** and **Colgate Orabase Soothe-N-Seal** form a long-lasting protective coating over the sore to speed healing and provide fast pain relief.

 A form of licorice known as **deglycyrrhizinated licorice, or DGL,** also coats canker sores. It's available in health-food stores. Chew one or two 200-milligram tablets two or three times a day.

 The sap of **aloe vera**—the ubiquitous "first aid plant"— can bring welcome relief. Squeeze a bit of gel from an aloe vera leaf. Dry the sore with a cotton swab, then dab on the gel. Repeat as often as you like.

 Cut open a **vitamin E** capsule and squeeze a bit of the liquid onto the sore.

Put It in Neutral

 Munch a chewable **Pepto-Bismol, Tums,** or **Rolaids** tablet or put it on the sore and allow it to dissolve. The pain you feel from a canker sore is caused by acids and digestive enzymes eating into the tissue in the sore. The tablets will neutralize the acids and may also speed healing. Check the label for dosage directions.

 Use a small amount of **milk of magnesia** as a mouth rinse, or apply it to the canker sore three to four times a day.

 Apply a damp **tea bag** to the sore for five minutes. Tea is alkaline, so it neutralizes acids. It also contains astringent compounds, which may help relieve the pain.

Get That Numb Feeling

🍂 Dab on a **topical anesthetic** such as **Anbesol** or **Orajel**.

🍂 Let a **pain-relieving lozenge**, such as **Chloraseptic**, dissolve in your mouth.

Battle Bacteria

🍂 Mix two ounces of **hydrogen peroxide** with two ounces of water. Add one teaspoon of **baking soda** and one teaspoon of **salt**, and stir until they dissolve. Swish the solution around in your mouth and spit it out. Hydrogen peroxide is a strong disinfectant. That's a plus, since a canker sore is an open wound that's vulnerable to infection, which increases the pain. And since baking soda is alkaline, it provides extra relief by neutralizing acids.

🍂 To speed healing, apply a liquid form of herbal **goldenseal** on the sore three times a day, at least an hour before eating. Goldenseal has modest antibacterial properties.

🍂 Put a single drop of **tea-tree oil**, an antiseptic, directly on the sore.

🍂 Make a tea from **calendula**, better known as pot marigold, valued for centuries in the treatment of minor sores. Pour a cup of boiling water over a teaspoon or two of dried petals. Let it steep for 10 minutes, strain out the leaves, and let the tea cool down until it's barely warm. You can gargle and rinse several times a day, or drink the tea.

🍂 Eat **yogurt** that contains live acidophilus cultures (check the label). Have a few teaspoonfuls daily for prevention—more when you're having a breakout.

Take Extra Measures

🍂 Many experts think **lysine**, an amino acid, may be needed to fix a deficiency associated with canker sores. Take 500 milligrams of L-lysine three times a day on an empty stomach until your sore is healed.

🍂 **Echinacea** is an herb that strengthens your immune system. Take 200 milligrams two or three times a day when you first notice a sore starting to appear.

🍂 **Vitamin C** helps heal your mouth's mucous membranes. Normally, we would turn to citrus fruits for vitamin C, but these may actually cause canker sores in some people. Instead,

Should I call **the doctor?**

If the pain is too distracting or it's keeping you from eating or drinking, call your dentist. Definitely call the dentist if you have more than four sores at a time or if the sores last longer than two weeks. Also, if you find that you're getting canker sores frequently, tell your dentist at your next visit so he or she can recommend evaluation and treatment, such as an antibiotic mouth rinse, a steroid ointment, a prescription oral paste, or chemical cautery of the sores.

take vitamin C supplements. Try 1,000 milligrams three times a day. If you develop diarrhea with dosages this high, switch to 500-milligram supplements instead.

🐭 **Zinc** may help mouth injuries like canker sores heal faster. As soon as you detect a sore developing, take 30 milligrams of zinc lozenges each day until it's gone.

The Power of Prevention

🐭 **Stay away from foods that trigger canker sores.** Potential troublemakers include whole wheat, rye, barley, shellfish, pineapple or citrus fruits, figs, chocolate, tomatoes, green peppers, and strawberries. To find out which, if any, cause your cankers, cut all of them out of your diet. Then slowly reintroduce them, one at a time, and see which one makes the problem recur.

🐭 Check the label of your favorite toothpaste for an ingredient called sodium lauryl sulfate, or SLS. This foaming agent, found in many brands of toothpaste, contributes to canker sores in some people. And it really isn't necessary for teeth cleaning. If you get frequent sores, **look for brands that are free of SLS** such as Biotene and Arm & Hammer Dental Care Tooth Powder.

🐭 Tiny cuts and scrapes inside your mouth can cause canker sores. **Take care when eating jagged foods** like chips and pretzels. When you brush your teeth, **use a soft-bristled brush** to avoid scraping your gums.

🐭 See your dentist if you have any kind of tooth problem that could irritate the inside of your mouth. **Ill-fitting dentures**, especially, can be a problem.

🐭 People plagued with frequent canker sores may have a deficiency in certain B vitamins or iron. Try taking a **daily B-vitamin complex** and a **daily multivitamin/multimineral** for iron. To get more B vitamins into your diet, look to beans, wheat germ, and fortified cereal. Lean beef is a good source of iron.

🐭 Stressful episodes trigger many cases of canker sores. If you tend to get a little wired, try some of the classic methods of keeping your cool—**meditation, yoga,** and **aerobic exercise.**

Carpal Tunnel Syndrome

The last time you needed a signed note from your doctor might have been senior year of high school. But if you now suffer from CTS, it may be time to ask your family physician for another one, because you need to play hooky from the activity that inflamed the tendons inside your carpal tunnel. Once you've got license to give wrists a respite, you can use splints, supplements, and exercises to help them recover. But even as you renew normal wrist action, take some preventive steps and keep up the strengthening exercises.

Get a Grip on the Pain

➤ To quickly ease the pain and inflammation, cool your wrists with an **ice pack** wrapped in a thin towel. Leave it on for about 10 minutes. You can repeat the treatment every hour or so.

➤ **Heat** can also ease pain by relaxing muscles. Soak your hands and wrists in warm to hot water for 12 to 15 minutes before you go to bed each night.

➤ Twice a day, rub your wrists with an ointment containing **arnica.** This herbal treatment, renowned for its anti-inflammatory properties, helps ease aches and pains. Dab the inside of each wrist with about one-quarter teaspoon of the ointment, then massage that area with the thumb of the other hand, all the way to the base of your palm. Repeat every morning and night until your symptoms ease.

➤ **Wear a splint at night.** While sleeping, you may be bending your hand and wrist under your pillow, and this puts pressure on your wrist. In fact, people with CTS are often awakened by the pain. A splint will hold your fingers in a neutral position and relieve pressure on the median nerve. You can purchase the splint in a medical supply store or pharmacy. But check with your doctor or physical therapist to make sure it fits properly.

➤ You may also want to **wear a splint during the day,** especially if you're doing jobs that require a lot of hand motion.

What's wrong

Inside each wrist is a narrow passageway called the carpal tunnel. Running through this tunnel are nine tendons that move your fingers, along with the median nerve. These tendons can become inflamed and swell, compressing the nerve. Repetitive hand motion is one well-known cause of carpal tunnel syndrome, but other factors include pregnancy, birth-control pills, rheumatoid arthritis, and being overweight. Among the symptoms are numbness or tingling in your thumb and first three fingers, pains that shoot up your wrist and forearm, soreness in the neck and shoulders, and hand weakness.

Should I call **the doctor?**

Seek a doctor's care if symptoms interfere with your daily activities. If CTS goes untreated, you could be left with weakened grip in your hands and significant pain in your forearms or shoulders. Also, the condition is associated with arthritis, diabetes, and underactive thyroid gland; a doctor needs to evaluate you to make sure you don't have one of those other conditions in addition to CTS.

Look for Supplemental Relief

Bromelain, an enzyme derived from pineapples, digests inflammatory proteins, so it can reduce inflammation in your sore wrists. Along with reducing the pain, it may help you heal faster. Bromelain's potency is measured in MCU (milk-clotting units) or GDU (gelatin-dissolving units). Look for supplements rated between 1,800 and 2,400 MCU or 1,080 and 1,440 GDU, and take 1,000 milligrams twice a day when you're having a CTS flare-up. You can cut down to 500 milligrams twice a day once your symptoms start resolving. Just be sure you take these supplements between meals. If you take them near mealtimes, much of their potency will be misspent digesting your food.

The herb **St. John's wort**, best known as an antidepressant, can also help repair nerve damage and reduce pain and inflammation. Take 150 to 250 milligrams of extract standardized to contain 0.3% hypericin three times a day. If that's not working after two weeks, take 300 to 400 milligrams three times a day.

Take a tablespoon of **flaxseed oil** every day, and give it at least two weeks to have an effect. Flaxseed oil is extremely rich in omega-3 fatty acids, which reduce inflammation. Take it with food for better absorption. If you like, you can mix it into your orange juice or add it to your salad dressing.

B for Benefit?

Vitamin B_6 is probably the most well-known supplement when it comes to treating carpal tunnel syndrome, but it's also controversial. Many experts claim it works, and many claim it doesn't. On top of that, excessive vitamin B_6 in the range of 1,000 to 2,000 milligrams a day can even *cause* nerve problems.

Supplementation with B_6 might be helpful, since the vitamin is important in maintaining healthy nerves, and it may speed up nerve impulses to your hands. Some people claim CTS is actually caused by vitamin B_6 deficiency. What we know for sure is that some people require more of the vitamin than others, and stress can increase your need for it.

To err on the side of caution, eat plenty of foods rich in the vitamin, including chicken breast, whole-grain cereals, brown rice, salmon, green vegetables, and egg yolks. If you want to try a supplement, take 50 milligrams of B_6 one to three times a day until your symptoms resolve, but do it under a doctor's supervision, especially if you take more than 100 milligrams a day.

✎ **Curcumin** is an anti-inflammatory component found in the spice turmeric. In Ayurvedic medicine—which originated in India—turmeric has a long history of use as a medicine for pain and inflammation. But the spice doesn't pack the punch of curcumin supplements. Take 300 milligrams three times a day of a supplement standardized to contain 95% curcumin.

✎ Try taking 300 milligrams of elemental **magnesium** two or three times a day. This trace mineral is involved in nerve function and muscle relaxation. A supplement may help, especially if you don't eat a lot of magnesium-rich whole grains, legumes, or green vegetables. The most absorbable forms are magnesium lactate, magnesium orotate, magnesium glycinate, and magnesium gluconate. The only side effect might be loose bowel movements. If you have that problem, just reduce the dose.

Take Precautions at the Keyboard

✎ If you spend a lot of time in front of the computer, **adjust your chair and keyboard.** Your arms should be bent at a 90-degree angle when you type so that your wrists are parallel with the ground. Knees, too, should obey the "90-degree rule." And sit up straight, making sure your shoulders aren't slumped forward.

✎ If the keyboard can be lowered, bring it down to a position where the **keys are slightly lower than your wrists** so that your fingertips drop down to rest lightly on the keys.

✎ **Tap the computer keys**, don't pound them. The less pressure you apply, the better.

✎ Use ergonomic, hand-friendly products whenever possible. Especially helpful is **a wrist rest**, sold at most office supply stores.

✎ Get a **contoured keyboard** or **split keyboard.** They are specially designed so your hands can rest in a natural position while your fingers tap lightly on the keys. (The pressure required to depress a key is much lighter than on regular keyboards.) In contour models, two sets of keys are held in a single, molded frame, with comfortable areas to support each of your wrists. Split keyboards have separate frames that can be angled in different ways for maximum wrist comfort.

Did you **know?**

Carpal tunnel syndrome didn't just start with the advent of widespread computer usage. You can get CTS from playing the piano, hammering in nails, or milking cows. Musicians, carpenters, and dairy farmers are all prone to CTS.

Chicken Pox

Chicken pox lasts only a week or two, but generally the end can't come soon enough. If pain is the problem, ease it with acetaminophen—never aspirin. If the itching is too much of a bear to bear, try cool baths and an antihistamine such as liquid Benadryl. And have a few other tricks to keep up your sleeve to minimize the misery.

What's wrong

Your child has a common childhood illness, caused by the varicella zoster virus. The virus debuts with the eruption of a rash and/or red spots on his back, chest, and belly, which spread to other areas within a few days. He may have a few spots or hundreds of them. Over a period of about a week, many of the spots turn into small blisters, which break and scab over. Your child may also have a fever and develop itching, which can be mild or intense. After the blisters heal, the virus goes into a latent stage and lives in sensory nerves in the body. It may surface years later in the form of the painful ailment shingles.

Stay Cool

 If it's winter, **turn down the heat** to the lowest comfortable temperature. In summer, use **air conditioning.** Heat brings more blood to the skin, which exacerbates the itch.

 Soak your child in a tub of slightly cool water for 15 to 20 minutes every few hours. Don't use soap. Instead, add one-half cup of **baking soda** to a shallow bath or one full cup to a deep bath to provide extra relief. **Colloidal oatmeal** (such as Aveeno) added to a bath also counteracts itching. If you don't have colloidal oatmeal, place regular oats in a nylon stocking, tie the end, and place the stocking in the water.

 Offer your child a **cool, wet washcloth** to press against her skin when she feels like scratching. Scratching can lead to infection and scarring. By using the washcloth, she'll satisfy the scratching urge without doing any damage. For insurance against scratching, keep her nails trimmed, and put her to bed with cotton gloves on her hands.

Attack the Itch

 Swab on some **calamine.** This over-the-counter lotion, made mostly of zinc oxide, helps by drying up the blisters.

 Try **bergamot oil.** Bergamot, which is derived from a citrus fruit closely related to the orange, is often used to flavor tea. But it has also been used for centuries in Italy to dry chicken pox blisters and relieve the itching. Bergamot is composed of 11% to 22% alcohols, which have a soothing, drying effect. Add 10 to 20 drops of bergamot essential oil to a carrier

Shun the Blistering Sun

If your child has recently been exposed to someone who has the chicken pox virus, keep her out of the sun. A dose of sunshine may make the blisters worse when they finally appear. After the chicken pox is over, your child's skin will remain sensitive to the sun for as long as a year. You don't have to barricade her in the house, but do apply sunscreen every day.

oil (such as olive oil, sweet almond oil, etc.) and mix well. Then apply to blisters.

➤ If the itching is bad, give your child an **oral antihistamine** such as **Benadryl.** Just be aware that it might make her drowsy.

Calm with Cotton

➤ Keep him in fresh **cotton PJs.** Cotton is less irritating than other fabrics. Make sure they have long sleeves and pants to discourage scratching.

Mind the Mouth

➤ If your child has chicken pox in his mouth (yes, it can happen), have him gargle with **salt water.**

➤ Give him **ice pops.** They can be soothing.

➤ Feed him **bland food** like Jell-O, soups, and bananas as long as the blisters are painful.

The Power of Prevention

➤ You can protect your child from chicken pox with a vaccine called **Varivax,** recommended for children one year and older who are in good health. The same vaccine is effective in adults who have never had chicken pox.

➤ If your child has not been vaccinated, you can prevent infection by keeping him away from other children who have chicken pox—but that may not be advisable. It is **far better to get chicken pox as a child.** The virus is much more serious in adults.

Should I call **the doctor?**

Chicken pox is usually more of an annoyance than a danger; most cases clear up in 10 to 14 days without problems. However, approximately 50 deaths related to chicken pox occur among children every year. Call your pediatrician if your child has a high fever accompanied by severe headache, has a fever that lasts more than a few days, feels severe pain in his limbs, repeatedly vomits, develops a cough, or has a large area of redness surrounding one or more blisters—a sign of infection. Also call your doctor if your child has convulsions, becomes disoriented, or complains that his neck hurts when he stretches it.

Cold Sores

Since the blisters come and go, the goal of every cold-sore veteran is to make sure they're absent a lot more than they're present. Once the virus is with you, you have to mount a constant campaign to keep it discouraged. However, you'll learn to recognize the telltale tingling or burning sensation that notifies you of a sore's imminent arrival, and if you're prepped ahead of time, you can pepper it with your defensive home remedies.

What's wrong

Cold sores are usually caused by the herpes simplex type I virus. The painful, fluid-filled blisters might appear on your lip, or you may have painful ulcers in your mouth and throat. If you get a sore once, you'll likely have a recurrence. A tingling sensation around your mouth heralds the sore's imminent arrival, usually within a day or two. The blister swells, bursts, oozes fluid, crusts over, and departs, often in 7 to 10 days. Painful sores on your tongue and inside your lips and cheeks may accompany an initial outbreak. Common triggers of a new outbreak include sunlight, stress, menstruation, and fatigue.

First Aid for Cold Sores

Apply **ice** directly to the sore. It will bring down the swelling and ease the pain temporarily. If you use this tactic early enough in the game—at the first sign of tingling—you may end up with a smaller sore than you otherwise would have.

You can also use **aspirin** for pain relief, and it may have an added benefit. The results of one study published in the *Annals of Internal Medicine* suggested that taking 125 milligrams of aspirin a day can cut the time a herpes infection remains active by 50 percent.

Vanquish the Virus

Time and again, the amino acid **lysine** emerges as the hands-down healer for cold sores. When you're having an outbreak, take 3,000 milligrams daily until the sore goes away. Research has shown that it thwarts the replication (copying) of the herpes virus.

Herbal healers commonly recommend **lemon balm** (also called melissa), which is used throughout Europe to treat herpes simplex 1. Its essential oils contain substances that have been shown to inhibit the virus. In German studies, people with recurrent cold sores who used a lemon balm ointment regularly had less frequent outbreaks, or stopped developing the sores altogether. Look for a lemon balm ointment in health-food stores, and use it as needed.

Dab the sore with a tincture of **myrrh** on a cotton swab up to 10 times a day. Myrrh directly attacks the virus that causes herpes. You'll find myrrh in health-food stores.

Blend **tea-tree oil** with an equal amount of **olive oil**, and apply it to the sore two or three times a day. Tea-tree oil is a powerful natural antiseptic. Research conducted in the 1920s showed it had up to 13 times the antiseptic power of carbolic acid, which was then a common germicide.

Eat **yogurt** that contains live acidophilus bacteria. Some studies have shown that the acidophilus bacteria found in some brands of yogurt actually hinder the growth of the virus.

Use an over-the-counter medication like **Abreva.** OTCs like this are most effective if you take them as soon as you feel the telltale tingle of an oncoming cold sore. The medication contains **docosanol**, which works by shielding healthy cells from those that have been infected by the virus. If taken immediately, the medication can shorten healing time by a day or so.

Bolster Your Defenses

During an outbreak, take one 300-milligram capsule of **echinacea** four times daily. Studies have shown that the herb can boost your immune system's ability to fight off the virus.

Take 1,000 milligrams of the immune-boosting flavonoid (plant pigment) **quercetin** each day in divided doses. Research published in the *Journal of Medical Virology* has shown that this supplement can speed the healing of cold-sore blisters. It's available in drugstores or health-food stores.

Don't Crack Up

After the sore has crusted over, coat it with some **petroleum jelly** to prevent it from cracking and bleeding. When you do this, however, make sure you don't transmit the virus to the stuff in the jar. Instead of using your finger, apply the petroleum jelly with a cotton swab. Use a fresh swab every time.

The Power of Prevention

If you get more than three cold sores a year, you might benefit from taking a daily **lysine** supplement as a preventive. The recommended dose is 500 milligrams a day.

Should I call **the doctor?**

Yes, if this is your first outbreak, if your sores last longer than two weeks, or if you get four or more cold sores a year. You may need the prescription antiviral drug acyclovir (Zovirax). Your doctor will also want to see you if your sore is accompanied by fever, swollen glands, or flulike symptoms, or if it's so painful that you avoid eating or brushing your teeth. Finally, if you develop eye pain or become sensitive to light, it may mean the virus has spread to your eyes. Get to a doctor quickly: Your vision may be in jeopardy.

Did you **know?**

Nearly all of us carry the cold-sore virus, even when it's not causing symptoms. An estimated 90 percent of adults age 40 and over carry herpes simplex I virus, the cause of most cold sores.

Since the virus that causes herpes is carried through saliva, some extra dental hygiene may be *de rigueur* to avoid recontaminating yourself after an outbreak.

 ➤ Keep your toothbrush in a dry spot, preferably on an open shelf where it's exposed to circulating air and sunlight. If that means keeping it outside the bathroom, so be it. A damp toothbrush in a moist bathroom is an invitation for viral breeding.

 ➤ Buy a small tube of toothpaste, use it during the outbreak, then throw it away.

 ➤ Replace your toothbrush after an outbreak.

Tried...

When nothing else was handy, folks used a dab of vinegar to head off a cold sore.

...and true

Vinegar is acidic, and viruses don't do well in an acidic environment. Use a cotton swab dipped in any kind of vinegar and apply to the affected area, repeating several times a day at the first suggestion of the telltale tingle. Throw the swab away after each use.

 ➤ **Stay away from** foods rich in **arginine**, an essential amino acid that the herpes virus needs in order to thrive. If you want to take maximum precautions to avoid an outbreak, **avoid chocolate, cola, beer, peas, nuts** (peanuts, cashews, almonds, and walnuts), **gelatin**, and **whole-grain cereals.**

 ➤ Take 15 milligrams of **zinc** each day. In test-tube studies, this nutrient has been shown to block the replication of the virus. Zinc also boosts the immune system and fortifies the surface tissue on your lips and on the inside of your mouth, making it difficult for the virus to take hold.

 ➤ Try to **avoid whatever seems to trigger outbreaks.** Do they appear after you've spent time in the sun, or during times of stress? Once you can pinpoint a likely cause, you can take measures to avoid setting the stage for new episodes.

 ➤ Use a **lip balm** that contains a sun protection factor (SPF) of at least 15. In one study of people with recurrent sores, those who didn't shield their lips were much more likely to develop blisters during extended exposure to sunlight.

 ➤ Like laughter and yawns, the sores are contagious. **Don't kiss your partner** if either of you has a cold sore. Direct contact with an infected person's saliva is usually necessary to pass the bug along, but if anyone in your house has cold sores, **don't mix up washcloths,** towels, drinking glasses, or toothbrushes.

 ➤ When you have a cold sore, **avoid touching your eyes.** Transmitting the virus to your eyes could cause a nasty infection that could potentially damage your eyesight.

Colds and Flu

It may be "just a cold," but it's nothing to sneeze at. And the flu can make you feel downright flattened. Fortunately, fast action on your part can mitigate the misery. Herbs, chicken soup, zinc —and even your blow-dryer—are part of the healing arsenal. At the first sign of a sniffle, turn to these remedies, which can unstuff your head, boost your immune engines, and speed your illness on its way—unlike typical cold medicines, which can dry you out, put you to sleep, keep you up at night, do nothing at all to make you better faster, and may even prolong your illness.

Think Zinc

At the first hint of a cold, suck on a **zinc gluconate** lozenge every few hours. In one study, people who sucked on one lozenge that contained about 13 milligrams of zinc every two hours while awake shook off their symptoms three to four days sooner than people who didn't. Don't take zinc gluconate longer than a week, though, because excessive zinc can actually weaken immunity. And avoid zinc lozenges that contain citric acid or are sweetened with sorbitol or mannitol; these ingredients seem to weaken the mineral's effectiveness.

Zicam, a nasal gel spray that contains zinc, may be even more effective than zinc lozenges. In a recent study at the Cleveland Clinic Foundation, people who used the gel saw their colds resolve in fewer than three days. Subjects who used a placebo had to wait nine days for their symptoms to go away.

Head Off a Head Cold

As soon as you notice cold or flu symptoms, start taking 500 milligrams of **vitamin C** four to six times a day. Buy a brand with added bioflavonoids, which have been shown to enhance the effectiveness of vitamin C by as much as 35 percent. If you develop diarrhea, cut down on the dose.

Take one 250-milligram **astragalus** capsule twice a day until you're better. This ancient Chinese herb stimulates the immune system and seems to be highly effective at fighting

What's **wrong**

If your symptoms are above the neck— congestion, sore throat, sneezing, coughing—you probably have a cold, caused by any one of 200 viruses that other people's sneezes or coughs have placed in the air or on something you've touched. If you have all those symptoms *plus* a fever of 102 degrees or more, headache, muscle aches, extreme fatigue, diarrhea, nausea, or vomiting, you're more likely to have the flu. The flu arises from one of three viruses, imaginatively named influenza A, B, and C. The flu can last from three to seven days.

Should I call **the doctor?**

Colds are miserable but generally go away on their own, speeded along by rest and home remedies. The same goes for mild cases of the flu; more severe cases may require a doctor's care. If you don't know which you have, let your symptoms be your guide. Your doctor will want to hear from you if you've had a fever above 101 degrees for more than three days, or any fever above 103 degrees. Call, too, if you start to wheeze, find it hard to breathe, feel severe pain in your lungs, chest, throat, or ear, or cough up copious amounts of sputum, especially if it's bloody or has a greenish tinge. For children, a fever can quickly lead to dehydration, so it's important to keep pushing fluids and to be in touch with your doctor.

colds and flu. To prevent a relapse, take one capsule twice a day for an additional week after your symptoms are gone.

🌿 **Goldenseal** stimulates the immune system and has germ-fighting compounds that can kill viruses. As soon as you begin to feel sick, take 125 milligrams five times a day for five days.

Bring On the Flu Fighters

🌿 At the first sign of the flu, take 20 to 30 drops of **elderberry** tincture three or four times daily for three days. Elderberry has been used in Europe for centuries to fight viruses, and research appears to bear out its effectiveness. In one study, people who took elderberry recovered faster from the flu than those who didn't. Ninety-three percent of the elderberry group saw their symptoms subside within two days, compared to six days in a group that didn't get the herb.

🌿 The homeopathic medicine Oscillococcinum, more commonly called **Oscillo**, is widely recommended by naturopaths, doctors, and herbalists to reduce the severity of flu symptoms. It is sold in most pharmacies and health-food stores. Be sure to use it within 12 to 48 hours of the first appearance of your symptoms. It comes in packages of three to six vials. Buy the three-vial pack and take one vial every six hours.

🌿 Try **N-acetyl cysteine (NAC)**, a form of the amino acid cysteine. It helps thin and loosen mucus and reduce flu symptoms. Take one 600-milligram dose three times daily.

Soothe a Sore Throat

🌿 For a sore throat, fill an 8-ounce glass with warm water, mix in 1 teaspoon of **salt**, and gargle away. The salt really does soothe the pain.

🌿 The traditional sore-throat gargle—a squeeze of **lemon juice** in a glass of warm water—is ideal because it creates an acidic environment that's hostile to bacteria and viruses.

Soup Up Your Cold-Fighting Engine

🌿 **Chicken soup**, that time-honored remedy of remedies, offers more than comfort for colds and flu. Modern scientists have confirmed that chicken soup stops certain white blood cells, called neutrophils, from congregating and causing inflammation, which in turn causes the body to produce copious amounts of mucus. It also thins mucus better than plain old hot water. Homemade soup is the best bet, especially if it's made by someone you love.

⌁ Add fresh chopped **garlic** to your chicken soup. The Egyptian pharaohs used garlic to fight infection, and its healing powers are legendary. Among its dozens of active compounds are allicin and allin, shown in test-tube studies to kill germs outright. The "stinking rose" also appears to stimulate the release of natural killer cells, part of the immune system's arsenal of germ-fighters.

Wet Your Whistle—and Everything Else

⌁ Fighting off colds and flu can rob your body of moisture. Drink as much **water** as you can—eight or more 8-ounce glasses—to keep your mucous membranes moist and to help relieve dry eyes and other common flu symptoms. Fluids also help thin mucus so that it's easier to blow it out.

⌁ To help keep mucus loose, stay in a **moist, warm, well-ventilated room.** To keep the air in your bedroom moist, place bowls of water near the radiator (in the winter) or run a humidifier.

A Reeking Remedy

⌁ A dose of **garlic**—a natural antiseptic—will do a job on those viruses. If you're feeling very brave, hold a small clove or a half-clove of garlic in your mouth and breathe the fumes into your throat and lungs. If it gets too strong as the clove softens, just chew it up quickly into smaller pieces and swallow with water.

Old **wives' tale**

Getting chilled does not cause a cold—at least not under laboratory conditions. In one study reported in *The New England Journal of Medicine*, two groups of people were exposed to viruses that cause the common cold. One group got their dose of germs in a 40-degree room; the other group, in a balmy 86-degree room. The result? Both groups caught colds at about the same rate.

Get a Shot at Staying Flu-Free

Consider getting a yearly flu shot (now also available as a nasal spray). Health authorities recommend it, especially for people with chronic heart or kidney disease, chronic lung diseases like asthma, bronchitis, emphysema, diabetes, or those with depressed immunity. It's also recommended for people over the age of 65. It takes 6 to 8 weeks for the shot to build up your immunity, so get vaccinated in the late fall, before the start of flu season.

Skip it!

Some cold medicines contain an antihistamine, which works well for allergies, but does nothing for congestion caused by colds. In fact, antihistamines can make mucus thicker and therefore harder to blow out or cough up. If you're stuffed up, choose a plain old decongestant. Pseudoephedrine is the ingredient least likely to cause side effects. If you use a nasal spray instead of a pill, don't use it for longer than two days; it can cause a rebound effect that makes your nose even stuffier.

You can also get a therapeutic dose of **garlic in capsule form.** Buy enteric-coated capsules, the kind that are easiest for the body to absorb. The typical dose is 400 to 600 milligrams four times a day, taken with food. Look for pills standardized to 4,000 micrograms of allicin potential.

Blow Away That Virus

You can cut short a cold with your...**blow-dryer?** As outlandish as it sounds, inhaling heated air may help kill a virus working its way up your nose. In one study conducted at Harvard Hospital in England, people who breathed heated air had half the cold symptoms of people who inhaled air at room temperature. Set your hair dryer on warm (not hot), hold it at least 18 inches from your face, and breathe in the air through your nose for as long as you can—at least 2 or 3 minutes, and preferably 20 minutes.

Clear Out Congestion

For a serious congestion-busting blast, buy fresh **horseradish** or **gingerroot**, grate it, and eat a small amount. (Alternatively, you can get the bottled forms of grated horseradish or ginger and eat as much as one-quarter to one-half tablespoon.) To guard against stomach upset, wait until after a meal to try this.

Drink a cup of **ginger tea.** Make it with a ginger tea bag or with one-half teaspoon of grated gingerroot. Ginger helps block the production of substances that cause bronchial congestion and stuffiness, and it contains compounds called gingerols, which are natural cough suppressants.

Spike broth or soup with a dash of **Tabasco sauce, red pepper flakes**, or **wasabi**, the condiment (usually made from horseradish) that's eaten with sushi. All of these red-hot add-ins can increase the broth's decongestant power. In fact, adding any of them to any food can help you breathe more freely.

Wear **wet socks** to bed. Believe it or not, this soggy strategy can help ease a fever and clear congestion by drawing blood to the feet, which dramatically increases blood circulation. (Blood stagnates in the areas of greatest congestion.) Best method: First warm your feet in hot water. Then soak a thin pair of cotton socks in cold water, wring them out, and slip them on just before going to bed. Put a pair of dry wool socks over the wet ones. The wet socks should be warm and dry in the morning, and you should feel markedly better.

~ Try soaking your feet in a **mustard footbath.** In a basin, mix 1 tablespoon of mustard powder in 1 quart of hot water. The mustard draws blood to your feet, which helps to relieve congestion.

~ An old-as-the-hills remedy for chest congestion involves a **mustard plaster** made from mustard seeds and flour or cornmeal. Grind up three tablespoons of mustard seeds and add the powder to a cup of flour or cornmeal. Stir in just enough water to make a paste, then slather it on your chest. The pungent aroma helps to unclog stuffy sinuses, and the heat improves blood circulation and eases congestion. Don't leave the plaster on for more than 15 minutes, however, or your skin may burn. You may want to smear on a bit of petroleum jelly before you apply the plaster to protect the skin.

Steam Clean Your Nasal Passages

~ Pour just-boiled water into a large bowl. Drape a towel over your head to trap the steam, and breathe in through your nose for 5 to 10 minutes. Don't lower your face too close to the water or you risk scalding your skin or inhaling vapors that are too hot.

~ To make steam inhalations even more effective, add 5 to 10 drops **thyme oil** or **eucalyptus oil** to the water. Keep your eyes closed as you breathe the steam, since both the essential oil and steam can be irritating to your peepers.

~ When you're on the go, dab some tissues with a few drops of **eucalyptus oil** and bring them with you. Whenever you feel congested, hold a tissue to your nose and inhale.

Ring a Stiff Neck

~ The flu can give you one doozy of a stiff neck. To take the ache away, wet a hand towel, wring it out, place it in a plastic bag, and **microwave it for 60 seconds.** Or simply **boil a towel in hot water.** The towel should steam when you remove it from the bag or the pot of water. When it's cool enough, wring it out. Then wrap the towel around your shoulders and neck and lie down. (Put a beach or bath towel under

Did you **know?**

When you blow your nose, do it gently. Otherwise you might create reverse pressure that can lead to the virus or bacteria going up into your sinuses. To keep the reverse pressure to an absolute minimum, blow one nostril at a time.

you to keep the bed or couch dry.) To lock in the heat, wrap a dry towel around the wet one.

The Power of Prevention

☙ During cold and flu season, take 20 to 30 drops of **echinacea** tincture in a half-cup of water three times a day. A tincture made with pure echinacea should cause a slight numbing sensation on your tongue. Take it for a few weeks, then wait a week before resuming.

☙ **Wash your hands often** with soap and warm water, especially after you use a public restroom or if you're around people who are sick. Don't touch your face with unwashed hands either. In 1998 the Naval Health Research Center conducted a study of 40,000 recruits who were ordered to wash their hands five times a day. The recruits cut their incidence of respiratory disease by 45 percent.

☙ Use a **humidifier** or **cool-mist vaporizer** during the winter months to keep indoor air moist.

☙ Practice **stress-control techniques** year-round, but especially during cold and flu season. Research suggests that the more stress you're under, the more likely you are to get sick.

☙ **Make love** at least once a week. In one study, men and women who were sexually active at least that often had higher levels of immune-system molecules called immunoglobulin A—which play an important role in shielding the mucous membranes from invaders—than people who weren't.

☙ **Get some rest.** Most people get colds and flus when they're run down. So call in sick and sleep. Research shows that even if you are marginally sleep-deprived, your resistance to viruses can decline dramatically. In one study, certain immune cells that stalk viral infections dropped by 30 percent in people who got just slightly less sleep than usual in a single night.

☙ **Widen your circle of friends.** In a study of over 200 men and women, people who had strong social ties developed fewer colds. Researchers gave the subjects nasal drops containing rhinovirus, the bug that causes most colds, and they found that those with only one to three social relationships were four times more likely to come down with a cold than those who had six or more friends.

Conjunctivitis

Conjunctivitis can itch. It can hurt. It can make you look like a beet-eyed alien. It can also injure your eyes, and if caused by bacteria or a virus, can spread like the plague. So what are you supposed to do? Start by seeking the help of a doctor. If you have an infection, he'll give you medicated eye drops that will speed healing and shorten contagion time. Meanwhile, you can take steps to ease the itch and control the crusting.

Get an Eyeful of Relief

➤ **Hot or cold compresses** can help. If you have a lot of discharge from your eyes, run a washcloth under warm water and use it as a compress to prevent the sticky secretions from drying on the lashes. Use a cold compress (soak a washcloth in ice water) to shrink swelling and reduce itchiness, especially if your conjunctivitis is caused by allergies. Do either one—or both—for five minutes three or four times a day. Use a fresh washcloth each time.

➤ Wipe away the secretions and crusty material with a cotton ball soaked in 1 part **baby shampoo** to 10 parts warm water. The warm water loosens the crust, and the shampoo cleans the area where your eyelid and eyelashes meet.

➤ Use an eyewash made of lightly **salted water.** Bring a pint of water to a boil, add 1 teaspoon of salt, and let it simmer for at least 15 minutes. Let the solution cool down. Use a sterile eyedropper or eyecup to apply the wash. After each treatment, sterilize the eyedropper or eyecup again in boiling water.

➤ A **goldenseal** eyewash will help fight infection. Goldenseal contains a compound called berberine that has antibacterial properties. To make the wash, steep one teaspoon of dried goldenseal in boiling water for ten minutes, strain, and let it cool. Apply with a sterile eyedropper three times daily.

Brace Yourself for Bed

➤ If your doctor has prescribed antibiotic or steroid **eye drops** or ointments, use them each night before you go to bed

What's **wrong**

When eyes are red, irritated, and glued shut with gummy secretions, you've probably got conjunctivitis. It's an inflammation of the conjunctiva, the transparent membrane that lines the inner eyelids and sheathes the globe of the eye. Commonly known as pinkeye, conjunctivitis is usually caused by a bacterial or viral infection or an allergic reaction to pollen, cosmetics, contact lens cleaning solution, or other substances. Depending on the type, conjunctivitis can cause your eyes to burn, itch, tear profusely, and become intensely sensitive to light. A sticky discharge glues your eyelashes and eyelids together while you sleep.

Should I call **the doctor?**

Mild cases of pinkeye, especially those caused by viruses, should go away on their own within a week. Still, some forms of the condition can lead to potentially serious eye damage, so call your doctor if your symptoms are severe. You will want to get your doctor's advice as soon as possible if your vision is blurred, if conjunctivitis doesn't go away on its own in a week, or if you don't see any improvement after 3 to 4 days of steady treatment. If you have bacterial conjunctivitis, quick treatment will prevent complications.

to ensure that your eyelids don't get "glued shut" while you sleep. Make sure the tip of the eyedrop bottle or tube does not touch your eyes. Otherwise, you might contaminate the medicine and potentially re-infect your eyes the next time you use it.

Soothers for Sore Eyes

Soothe your eyes with a **chamomile** compress. Place a chamomile tea bag in warm (not hot) water for 2 to 3 minutes, squeeze out the excess liquid, then place the tea bag over your sore eye or eyes for 10 minutes. Repeat three or four times a day with a fresh tea bag. Keep your eyes closed so the wash doesn't come into direct contact with your eye.

Practitioners of Ayurveda, the traditional medicine of India, treat conjunctivitis with the pulp of fresh **cilantro** leaves. In a blender or chopper, blend a handful of cilantro leaves with one-quarter to one-third cup water. Strain out the juice, and apply the pulp to your closed eyelids. Leave it on for a few minutes, then wipe away the mixture before you open your eyes.

Another Ayurvedic treatment is to steep 1 teaspoon of **coriander** seeds in 1 cup of boiling water for at least 15 minutes. Strain thoroughly, cool, and use the water to bathe your closed eyes. Wipe away the excess before you open your eyes.

Contain the Contagion

To avoid re-infection of one or both eyes, **don't wear eye makeup or contact lenses** until the infection is com-

Three Types of Pinkeye

The three most common types of conjunctivitis are viral, bacterial, and allergic. Because there is some overlap of symptoms, you will need a doctor's diagnosis to distinguish one from the other. However, here are the characteristic signs of each kind:

VIRAL
- Infection usually begins with one eye, but may spread to the other
- Watery discharge
- Irritation/redness

BACTERIAL
- Usually affects only one eye, but may spread to the other
- Irritation, redness, and/or a gritty feeling
- Copious discharge

ALLERGIC
- Usually affects both eyes
- Itching and tearing
- Swollen eyelids

pletely gone. Throw away any eye makeup you were using when the infection developed.

~ **Try not to touch your eyes.** If you touch them accidentally, wash your hands with soap and water, then dry with a paper towel or hot-air dryer instead of a hand towel.

~ If you have to dab your eyes, use a **separate tissue** for each eye. Immediately throw both tissues in a plastic bag and wash your hands. When it's time to throw out the plastic bag, do it yourself and wash your hands thoroughly afterward.

~ Carry a small bottle of **antibacterial hand gel** with you and use it often.

~ If you wear **contact lenses, clean and sterilize them** exactly according to the manufacturer's directions, whether or not you or anyone around you shows signs of conjunctivitis. Wash your hands before you put in or take out your lenses. And never, ever clean a contact with saliva.

~ At home, after you eat, **put your dishes and utensils in the dishwasher yourself.** Don't let anyone else handle them.

~ Throw your towel, washcloth, and pillowcase **into the laundry** every day. This helps prevent you from re-introducing the bacteria or virus to the same eye or spreading it to the other eye. (Also, other people can pick up infectious conjunctivitis by using the same washcloth or towels that you've been using.)

~ **Let someone else make the bed.** Conjunctivitis can be spread from your hands to the sheets.

~ If you have young children with conjunctivitis who are too young to follow the rules about not touching their eyes and washing their hands, they should **stay home from school.**

For Allergic Conjunctivitis

~ If your eye itches and produces a stringy discharge, your conjunctivitis may be the result of allergies. Try taking an **oral antihistamine** to relieve the itching and swelling.

~ To help combat inflammation caused by allergies, try a combination of **vitamin C** and **quercetin.** Take 1,000 milligrams a day of vitamin C in divided doses, together with 1,500 milligrams of quercetin. Quercetin is one of a class of nutrients called bioflavonoids—derived from a wide range of fruits and vegetables—that have anti-inflammatory properties.

Skip it!

Some herbal healers recommend eyebright to treat conjunctivitis, based on its traditional use among Native Americans for relieving eye problems. However, recent studies have shown that eyebright can actually cause tearing, itching, and redness if it comes in contact with the eye. Its therapeutic value has never been proved.

Constipation

Your first instinct when you're in this predicament might be to reach for a laxative. But chances are you don't need one. The best way to get "regular" again is simply to eat more fiber—20 to 35 grams a day. Fiber absorbs water and makes your stool softer and larger, which speeds it through your system. To cope with all that fiber, you'll need more fluids too. And don't forget about exercise, which can also help keep things moving. Do all three things and you'll certainly put a smile back on your face instead of that, well, constipated look.

What's wrong

You hear nature's call, and you want to answer, desperately. But your body won't respond—or when it does, your stools are hard, dry, and difficult or painful to pass. The most common reason bowels go on strike is because you lack fiber or water in your diet. But there are other possible causes, such as lack of exercise, using laxatives or enemas too often, and health conditions such as diabetes, hypothyroidism, severe depression, or irritable bowel syndrome. Certain prescription or nonprescription medications may be culprits as well.

Fix It with Fiber

▸ Start your day with a **high-fiber bran cereal**. Some brands contain as much as 14 grams of insoluble fiber, the kind that adds bulk to stool, which spurs the body to move it through the digestive tract more quickly. A word to the wise: If you're not used to eating this much fiber, start with a smaller serving—say, one-quarter cup, served with skim milk or low-fat yogurt—then work your way up. Otherwise you may experience gas, bloating, and cramps.

▸ Fill up on cooked **dried beans, prunes, figs,** and **oatmeal.** All are rich in soluble fiber, the kind that turns to gel in the intestines and helps to soften stool. Pears are also good sources of soluble fiber.

▸ Mix one to two teaspoons **psyllium** seeds into a cup of hot water. Let it sit for two hours, add lemon and honey to taste, then drink. Psyllium adds bulk to stool and is the main ingredient in many OTC bulk-forming laxatives. You'll find the seeds in most drugstores and health-food stores. You can also try this remedy with flaxseeds.

▸ **Flaxseeds** are high in fiber and also contain heart-healthy omega-3 fats. Take 1 tablespoon of the ground seeds, which are sold in health-food stores, two or three times a day. Some people like the taste of flaxseed (it faintly resembles walnuts). If you don't, you can hide it in your morning cereal, stir it into applesauce, or add it to a fruit smoothie. Or grind the seeds in a spice grinder or coffee grinder, keep the ground-up seeds in the fridge, and sprinkle a half-teaspoon into your orange juice.

🍂 As you increase your intake of fiber, also be sure to drink **lots of water**—at least eight 8-ounce glasses a day. Fiber is extremely absorbent, and when you don't drink enough, your stools may become small, hard, and painful to pass.

Have a Hot Cup to Loosen Up

🍂 Have a morning cup of joe. If you're a java drinker, you may have already discovered that the **caffeine** in coffee has a bowel-loosening effect. It induces a bowel movement by stimulating the colon. Just don't drink too much of it—caffeine is a diuretic and will eliminate fluid from your body.

🍂 If you don't like coffee, try any other **hot beverage** first thing in the morning. Herbal or decaffeinated tea or a cup of hot water with a little lemon juice or honey may stimulate the colon as well. (Lemon juice is a natural laxative.)

🍂 **Dandelion tea**, which has a mild laxative effect, may help to get you regular again. Steep 1 teaspoon dried root in 1 cup boiling water and drink one cup three times a day. You'll find the dried dandelion root in health-food stores.

Wrinkle Your Nose—but It Works

🍂 One of Mom's favorite remedies, **castor oil**, really does help relieve constipation. A component in the oil breaks down into a substance that stimulates the small and large intestines. Take 1 to 2 teaspoons on an empty stomach, and give it 8 hours to do its work.

Wrinkled Fruit Works Too

🍂 The humble **prune** is one of the oldest home remedies for constipation. It's high in fiber (three prunes contain 3 grams

Should I call **the doctor?**

Although bothersome, constipation is usually not grave. However, it can sometimes signal a serious condition such as colorectal cancer or bowel obstruction. Tell your doctor if it lasts two weeks or more even when you're following the recommendations in this chapter. And call your doctor immediately if you see blood in your stool or if constipation is accompanied by fever, severe abdominal pain, or cramps. Also, if you've recently started a new medication that seems to cause constipation, you'll want to talk to your doctor. Possible drug culprits include antihistamines, diuretics, blood-pressure drugs, sedatives, calcium supplements, certain antidepressants, and antacids that contain calcium or aluminum.

Constipation—Reality or Illusion?

The advertising world would have us believe that daily elimination is the pinnacle of perfect health. Untrue, say doctors. Many of us fall prey to what they call "perceived constipation"—that is, we think we're constipated, but our bodies don't. People have varying body rhythms, and it's just as healthy (for some people) to go once every three days as it is (for others) to go three times a day.

Fiber All-Stars

If you're wondering how to get more fiber in your diet for better regularity, look to these foods, all excellent sources of soluble and insoluble fiber.

Food	Portion Size	Grams of Fiber	Food	Portion Size	Grams of Fiber
Bran cereal	½ cup	10–14	Pinto beans, canned	½ cup	5.5
Raspberries	1 cup	8.4	Lima beans,		
Red kidney beans, canned	½ cup	8.2	frozen, cooked	½ cup	5.4
Shredded Wheat			Oatmeal, cooked	1 cup	5.0
'N Bran cereal	1¼ cups	7.9	Green split-pea soup	1 cup	5.0
Lentils, boiled	1½ cups	7.8	Pears, raw	1	4.0
Blackberries	1 cup	7.6	Almonds	1 ounce	3.3
Black beans, boiled	½ cup	7.5	Prunes, canned	5	3.3
Figs, dried	3	6.9	Pearl barley, cooked	½ cup	3.0
Navy beans, canned	½ cup	6.7	Dates	5	3.0
Whole-wheat spaghetti,			Prunes, dried	5	3.0
cooked	1 cup	6.3			

of fiber). Also, prunes contain a compound called dihydroxyphenyl isatin, which stimulates the intestinal contractions that make you want to go.

➤ Don't like prunes? Open a box of **raisins.** They, too, are high in fiber and contain tartaric acid, which has a laxative effect. In one study in which people ate 4½ ounces (one small box) of raisins a day, doctors determined that it took half the time for digested food to make it through the digestive tract.

Get Up and Go

➤ Get regular **exercise.** There's a reason a daily walk is called a daily constitutional. When you move your body, you also help move food through your bowel more quickly. Aim for a daily walk at the very least.

Put the Pressure On

➤ One of the more unusual remedies for constipation is **acupressure.** Practitioners of this technique say that it helps stimulate your digestion—and, therefore, your bowels. Apply pressure with your thumb to the point four finger-widths above your wrist on the back of the forearm. Do this for two minutes every day while the problem persists.

Last Resorts

The herb **cascara sagrada** is so effective it's even added to several over-the-counter laxatives. It's known as a stimulant laxative because it stimulates the intestinal tract. The herb comes in a variety of forms; follow the dosage directions on the package. But don't take it for more than two weeks; it can make your body lose too much fluid and salt—and with habitual use, you can become dependent on it.

If other remedies fail to bring relief, try the mother of all natural laxatives: **senna.** It should work in about 8 hours, so most people take it before bedtime. Take 20 to 40 drops of the tincture at night, but don't plan on making it a long-term cure. With repeated use, it can cause cramps and diarrhea. As with cascara sagrada, long-term use can cause dependency.

Final Pointers

Never try to **force a bowel movement.** You may give yourself hemorrhoids or anal fissures. These not only hurt, they aggravate constipation because they narrow the anal opening.

Never ignore nature's call. If you do, you're asking for a case of constipation.

Coughs

Coughing not only annoys you but also makes you persona non grata at the movies, the symphony, and any other place where people congregate. But if you have a "wet" cough, you don't want to suppress it; that's because it's the body's way of clearing out mucus. Rather, you actually want to encourage it so you can get rid of the phlegm faster and get the coughing over with. If you have a "dry" cough, on the other hand, the trick is to coat the throat and tame the tickle.

What's **wrong**

Most likely, a cold or the flu is the cause of your hacking. An infection of the upper respiratory tract can cause swelling and irritation of the upper airways and, at times, mucus, which you cough up as phlegm. There are two kinds of coughs. A wet, or productive, cough, which yields mucus, is usually caused by allergies, colds, or other respiratory infections. A dry, or unproductive, cough may also be caused by a cold but is more often caused by cigarette smoke, dust, fumes, or some other form of irritation. This cough does nothing but irritate your throat, making you hack more.

Take the Candy Cure

For "wet" coughs, suck on **horehound candy**, available in drugstores. A bittersweet herb, horehound acts as an expectorant, triggering the coughing reflex and helping bring up phlegm.

For "dry" coughs, rely on **slippery elm lozenges.** Made from the bark of the slippery elm tree, these were once medicine-chest staples. Slippery elm is loaded with a gel-like substance that coats the throat and keeps coughing to a minimum.

No slippery elm lozenges? For a dry cough, any hard candy will do because it increases saliva and causes you to swallow more, suppressing coughs. **Lemon drops** work especially well for "wet" coughs.

Another remedy calls for combining **peppermint candy, lemon juice,** and **honey.** Heat the candy in lemon juice until the latter is dissolved. Then add honey and stir. Take 1 to 2 tablespoons as needed.

Dose a Cough with Down-Home Syrups

Blend **lemon juice** with a little **honey**, then add a pinch of **cayenne pepper** and swallow. The honey coats your throat, soothing irritated tissues, while the lemon reduces inflammation and delivers a dose of infection-fighting vitamin C. The red pepper increases circulation to the area, which hastens the healing process.

A very simple cough syrup calls for 2 tablespoons **lemon juice** and 1 tablespoon **honey.** Heat until warm and take as many teaspoons as you need, Add a bit of grated onion for a stronger kick. Onions contain irritating compounds that trigger the cough reflex and bring up phlegm.

🌿 Peel and finely chop 6 medium **onions.** Put them, along with a half-cup **honey,** into the top of a double boiler or in a pan over a pot of boiling water. Cover and let simmer for 2 hours. Strain and pour the mixture into a covered jar. Take 1 tablespoon every 2 to 3 hours.

🌿 For a throat-soothing syrup, mix 5 or 6 **cloves** with 1 cup **honey** and leave the mixture in the refrigerator overnight. In the morning, remove the cloves and take 1 teaspoon or 1 table-spoon of the honey as needed. Cloves dull the pain of a sore throat, while honey soothes inflamed throat tissues.

🌿 **Rock candy,** made from crystallized sugar, and one of the oldest forms of candy, is the basis of several old-time cough syrups. One recipe combines 1 box rock candy, 1 pound raisins, the juice of 3 lemons, one half-cup sugar, and enough whiskey to form a syrup. Another calls for 1 pound rock candy, 4 jiggers brandy, a half-jar honey, and the juice of 3 lemons. You'll have to make either recipe ahead of time, as it takes a few weeks for the rock candy to dissolve.

🌿 For a tasty old-time cough syrup, slice 3 **lemons** and place them in a pan with **honey** and a bit of **horehound** leaves and flowers. Horehound, a bitter herb once popular in cough "candies," acts as an irritant to trigger the cough reflex and bring up phlegm. Simmer the concoction until the syrup thickens. Strain the syrup and let it cool.

Brew Up a Cough-Taming Tea

🌿 **Thyme** is an expectorant and also contains substances that relax the respiratory tract. To make thyme tea, place

Should I call **the doctor?**

Most coughs clear up on their own within a week to 10 days. But if yours lasts more than 2 weeks, or you cough up blood, make the call. Coughing can be a symptom of a more serious illness, such as chronic obstructive pulmonary disease (COPD) and asthma. It can even indicate congestive heart failure, especially if it's accompanied by wheezing, shortness of breath, or swelling of the legs. If you have sharp chest pains, chills, or a fever higher than 101 degrees as well as a cough, you may have pneumonia.

Steam Away the Croup

A child with croup has a barking cough that often worsens at night. Caused by a viral or bacterial infection, croup is not usually dangerous, but it can be extremely frightening to parents. To treat it, take your child into the bathroom and run a hot, steamy shower. Keep him in the steam until the croup subsides. If it doesn't improve— or if the child is struggling to breathe—call your doctor or take him to the emergency room.

If your cough kicks up mainly after meals, at night, or while lying down, your problem might not be in your chest but in your stomach. Heartburn results when stomach acids back up into your lower esophagus, irritating the delicate tissue—which can lead to coughing. If you deal with heartburn symptoms (see page 140), you may find that you take care of the cough as well.

2 tablespoons fresh thyme (1 tablespoon dried) in a cup of hot water. Allow it to steep, then drain out the herb, add honey if you like, and drink.

 ᴖ Sip a cup of **marshmallow tea.** When combined with water, marshmallow yields a gooey mucilage that coats the throat and also thins mucus in the lungs, making it easier to cough up. To make the tea, steep 2 teaspoons of the dried herb in one cup hot water. Have a total of three cups a day.

 ᴖ Add 45 drops of **licorice** tincture to a cup of hot water and sip. Licorice loosens phlegm and relaxes bronchial spasms. A caution: Don't take licorice for more than a few weeks, as it can raise blood pressure.

 ᴖ Steep 2 teaspoons **horehound leaves or flowers** in 1 cup boiling water, strain, and drink.

 ᴖ Practitioners of Ayurveda, the traditional medicine of India, recommend a spice tea that you can drink several times a day. To make the tea, add a half-teaspoon powdered **ginger** and a pinch each of **clove** and **cinnamon** powder to a cupful of just-boiled water and drink.

Rub On Relief

 ᴖ Buy a **chest rub** that contains **camphor** or **menthol** and apply it to your throat and chest. Both of these substances have been FDA-approved as topical antitussives, which simply means they stop a cough. They should not be taken internally.

 ᴖ If you don't have any store-bought chest rub, try making a **mustard plaster** to loosen up chest congestion. Mix one part mustard powder and two parts flour in a bowl. Add just enough water to make a paste. Spread the paste on a dishtowel, fold the towel in half, and press it against the skin. (Never put the mustard mixture directly on your skin.) Check your skin often and remove the plaster if your skin becomes too red or

Choosing a Cough Syrup

When you're staring at a drugstore shelf jammed with cough elixirs, which one do you choose? If you're bringing up phlegm, buy an expectorant cough syrup (one that contains guaifenesin) to take during the day. It will loosen up the mucus and help you expel it. Only take a cough suppressant (look for codeine or dextromethorphan on the label) if you have a dry cough. Don't buy any cough syrup that contains both an expectorant and a cough suppressant—believe it or not, some do! As an alternative to these cough syrups, try Chestal syrup by Boiron. It's a cough preparation recommended by homeopathic doctors, and has no unwanted side effects.

irritated. Some people suggest using an egg white instead of water to make a plaster that's less likely to burn.

Learn a New Coughing Technique

If your throat is strained and irritated from nonstop coughing, try this technique to head off a coughing fit. The next time you feel a cough coming on, **force yourself to take a series of small, gentle coughs**, finally ending with a large one. The tiny coughs help move mucus toward the upper part of your air passage so you can expel more of it with that last, big cough.

Put Some Rhythm in Your Remedy

If you're at home and you have a partner who can help, use a chest-percussion technique to help clear chest congestion. Lie on your stomach on a firm bed or mat. Ask your partner to **slap cupped hands rhythmically** over the back, progressing from the lower back up toward the neck. Repeat several times until your congestion starts to loosen up.

Lights Out, Vapor On

To help prevent nocturnal coughing, use a **humidifier** in your room to moisten the air, particularly in winter.

Cuts and Scrapes

If you can stop the bleeding and keep the wound clean to prevent infection, you've done your part; nature will take over from there. Required: some bandages and antibiotic ointment (doctors recommend any triple antibiotic variety). Other wound remedies that work in a pinch are within easy reach—from honey to garlic to your own saliva.

What's wrong

You have just sliced yourself with a sharp object—a kitchen knife, your razor, a broken drinking glass, even a piece of paper. Or you've had a sudden encounter with a section of concrete and lost a bit of skin on your elbow or knee. There may be visible bleeding—and perhaps an invisible invasion of bacteria into the wound, bringing a risk of infection.

Clean, Cover, and Disinfect

➤ To stanch bleeding, apply **pressure** to the wound with a clean cloth or piece of gauze. In a pinch, use your hand.

➤ Once bleeding has stopped, gently clean the area around the wound with soap and water. Then apply a bandage.

➤ You can also cleanse a cut with a tincture of **calendula**, a bacteria-slaying herb known for its wound-healing powers. Look for calendula succus, which is a low-alcohol formula. If you can't find it, use the regular tincture and dilute it with a little water. To heal scrapes faster, try a calendula cream, sold in some health-food stores.

➤ Twice a day, you can clean your cut with **myrrh**, which stimulates the production of white blood cells. These are the infection-fighting cells that gather at the wound site. Mix 1 teaspoon myrrh tincture (available at health-food stores) with 4 ounces water. Dribble it over the cut or scrape, and allow the wound to remain exposed to the air until it dries.

➤ Try **tea-tree oil.** It contains a strong antiseptic compound and is popular the world over for treating wounds. Stir 1½ teaspoons of the oil into a cup of warm water and use this to rinse cuts and scrapes.

Cures from Your Kitchen

➤ No antibiotic cream handy? In a pinch, dab on a little **honey** and then cover with a bandage. Honey has antibacterial properties, and studies have shown that it can speed wound healing. In certain cases some doctors believe that honey might even be superior to triple-antibiotic creams as a wound dressing. Don't have a Band-Aid? Don't worry—honey dries to form a natural one.

🌿 **Garlic** is another of nature's antibiotics. Try taping a crushed clove over the cut. If it irritates your skin, take it off right away.

Scraped Knee? Bag It

🌿 It seems like kids manage to scrape their knees every day. Solution: **Bag Balm.** Originally designed for use on cows' udders, it protects scraped skin and keeps scabs soft so that they're less tempting to pick at. Vaseline, or any other kind of **petroleum jelly**, is also effective.

Take a Lesson from Rover

🌿 If you can't wash a wound—say you're smack in the middle of the woods—**lick it.** Researchers at the National Institute of Dental and Craniofacial Research demonstrated that a protein in saliva not only helps to heal wounds, it also acts as an anti-inflammatory, antiviral, antifungal, and anti-°bacterial agent.

Glue It Together

🌿 Read the warning label on **Instant Krazy Glue**, and you'll learn that it "bonds skin instantly." But if you've got a very small slice in your finger (like a paper cut), maybe an instant skin-sealer is just what you want. In fact, Krazy Glue contains the same ingredients as a new "liquid Band-Aid," and just a drop on a cut will seal it closed for quicker healing. Just make sure you don't touch that drop while it's drying, or you'll end up with a very awkward case of Siamese fingers.

Should I call **the doctor?**

Call the doctor if your wound won't close or stop bleeding, or if you have any signs of infection, (pus, unusual discharge, fever, red streaks that spread outward from the wound). If you have a deep puncture wound, your doctor may insist that you get a tetanus booster.

Tried...

Some people claim that pouring black pepper on a cut will stop the bleeding in a snap.

...and true

It may or may not stop the bleeding any faster, but black pepper does have painkilling, antiseptic, and antibiotic properties.

Dandruff

Do your shoulders look as if you just walked in from a snowstorm? Are you blinded by a blizzard every time you comb your hair? Dandruff isn't a serious health problem, but it sure can be embarrassing. To factor out those flakes, use the right shampoo. You can also whip up a homemade scalp rinse that will beat the yeast behind many cases of dandruff and give the dreaded itch the axe.

What's wrong

Like snakes, we humans continually shed outer layers of dead skin. When those skin cells slough off the scalp at turbo speed, you have yourself a case of dandruff. The condition has many possible causes. Stress is one. Others include overactive oil glands and seborrheic dermatitis—an itchy, scaly rash that can affect the face and chest as well as the scalp. There's evidence to suggest that dandruff is often caused by an overgrowth of a common yeast, called *Pityrosporum orbiculare*. The yeast feeds on skin oils—which may explain why people who have oily scalps are more susceptible to dandruff.

Wash Dandruff Away

⤙ Look for shampoos with **selenium sulfide, tar,** or **zinc pyrithione,** such as Denorex Enriched Formula Dandruff Shampoo. Anti-dandruff shampoos with these ingredients retard the rate at which scalp cells multiply. They are more effective than products formulated with sulfur or salicylic acid, such as Neutrogena T/Sal Therapeutic Shampoo, which loosen flakes so they can be washed away.

⤙ If your dandruff doesn't respond to a shampoo like Denorex, try one that contains **ketoconazole,** such as Nizoral. Ketoconazole is an antifungal medication that will kill the yeast that may be causing your dandruff.

⤙ If your dandruff shampoo stops working after a few months, your scalp probably got "used to" the active ingredient and started to "ignore" it. Just switch to a shampoo made with a **different active ingredient.** You may need to switch back in another few months.

⤙ Leave on dandruff shampoo for **at least 10 minutes** before you rinse to let it do its best work. For a serious case of flakes, lather up, plunk a shower cap on your head, and leave the shampoo on for an hour. You might want to extract a promise from your spouse or significant other not to laugh.

Rely on Rinses

⤙ Make a dandruff rinse using the herb **goldenseal**. It contains berberine, which has strong antibacterial and antifungal properties. Pour 1 cup of boiling water over 2 teaspoons of chopped root. Steep, strain, and let it cool. Use it as a rinse after you've shampooed, or any time during the day. If you can't find goldenseal root, add a few drops of goldenseal tincture to a little bit of shampoo.

Brew up a fragrant **rosemary** rinse. Like goldenseal, rosemary fights bacteria and fungi. And rosemary is a lot easier to find. To make the rinse, pour 1 cup of boiling water over 1 teaspoon of chopped rosemary. Let it sit for a few minutes, then strain. Use the liquid as a rinse once a day. If the rinse irritates your skin, move on to a different remedy.

Another herbal anti-dandruff rinse is made with **bay leaves**. Add a handful of crushed bay leaves to a quart of very hot (just boiled) water. Cover and let steep for 20 minutes. Strain, allow to cool, and apply. You might want to leave it in your hair for an hour or so before rinsing.

Apple cider vinegar, which kills a variety of fungi and bacteria, is frequently recommended as a home remedy for dandruff. Mix one part water with one part apple cider vinegar. Apply as a rinse after you shampoo.

Try Tea Tree

Tea-tree oil has strong antifungal properties. Dilute the oil in a little bit of a carrier oil (such as olive or grape-seed oil) and apply to your scalp. Leave it overnight. Or add a few drops to your shampoo. In health-food stores you may find shampoos with tea-tree oil already in them.

A Cultured Cure

It's not pretty, but it may work: Spread **yogurt** on your scalp and leave it there for half an hour, then rinse. Yogurt contains "friendly" bacteria that keep yeast in check. That's why it's also a traditional remedy for yeast infections.

Get the Flax

Take 1 to 2 teaspoons of **flaxseed oil** a day. It contains essential fatty acids, which seem to help itchy skin conditions such as psoriasis and eczema—and possibly dandruff. Be patient; you may need to take it for up to 3 months to see a difference. A side benefit: Flaxseed oil also helps guard against heart disease.

Should I call **the doctor?**

Normally, a mild case of dandruff will respond to self-treatment, so give home remedies or OTC dandruff shampoos about two weeks to work. Call your doctor if there's no improvement or if you have severe itching along with a red, irritated scalp. You'll also want a doctor's advice if you notice thick scaling, yellowish crusting, or red patches along your neckline. These symptoms suggest seborrheic dermatitis, a condition that requires medical advice and treatment.

Depression

What did Ludwig van Beethoven, Winston Churchill, and Vincent van Gogh have in common? They all, at one time or another, suffered from depression. In fact, depression is so widespread that some psychologists call it the common cold of emotional disorders. If you're depressed, you're not alone. Neither do you have to let depression control your life. For severe, chronic depression, there are effective prescription medications as well as various forms of therapy. For mild to moderate depression that comes and goes, there are plenty of depression-busting strategies you can implement on your own.

What's wrong

Maybe you've experienced a traumatic event. Or maybe, for no reason you can put your finger on, you just feel sad and empty. Depression is usually linked to a combination of medical, genetic, and environmental factors. There are four types: major depression, in which the emotional low is severe and lasts for more than two weeks; mild depression, or dysthymia, which has milder or fewer symptoms; bipolar disorder, which causes extreme mood swings; and postpartum depression, which sometimes happens to a mother after giving birth.

Work It Out

~ Get out there and move your body. Numerous studies have confirmed that **frequent exercise** can be a powerful mood enhancer. For mild or moderate depression it may even work as well as antidepressants. All you need is at least 20 minutes' worth of aerobic exercise three times a week. Walk, lift weights, jump rope, cycle—any form will do. Work up a sweat to get the best effect.

Look to Food to Change Your Mood

~ If you're on a high-protein diet for weight loss, **lack of carbohydrates** could be contributing to your blue mood. Foods like fruits and vegetables, beans, and whole grains help your brain make the mood-regulating brain chemical serotonin.

~ Aim to **eat fish** three times a week or more. Researchers in Finland found that people who ate fish less than once a week had a 31 percent higher incidence of mild to moderate depression than people who ate fish more often. Albacore tuna, salmon, sardines, and mackerel are top choices; they're rich in omega–3 fatty acids, essential to normal brain function. There's preliminary evidence that they influence serotonin production.

~ If you drink **coffee** or **cola**, cut back or even **give it up**. Research links caffeine, which suppresses serotonin production, to depression.

▲ **Nix alcohol**. While wine, beer, or hard liquor may initially raise spirits, alcohol is actually a depressant.

Put It in Writing

▲ **Record your feelings** on paper—especially painful feelings. Research shows that people who write about their most painful emotions for 20 minutes a day dramatically improve their psychological well-being after just four days. Sit with a blank piece of paper in front of you and write nonstop about the most distressing event in your life right now. Don't think; just write.

Lift Your Spirit

▲ **Attend services** at your church or temple. In a study of 4,000 older people, researchers found that those who frequently attended worship services were half as likely to be depressed as those who didn't.

Down a Mood Lifter

▲ Take 1,600 milligrams daily of **SAM-e**, pronounced "Sammy." In many European countries, the effectiveness of SAM-e against depression is so well accepted that the supplement is often prescribed by doctors for it. SAM-e is a naturally occurring substance found in every living cell. Low levels have been linked with depression. Dozens of studies have shown that SAM-e produced significant improvement after three weeks. In animal studies, SAM-e was found to boost the levels of three neurotransmitters—serotonin, dopamine, and norepinephrine—involved in mood changes. Some doctors point out that the form most often sold in the United States—tosylate disulfate—is highly unstable, and is only effective if it's taken in enteric-coated capsules. The preferred form is butanedisulfonate, which can be ordered from Nature Made and GNC. Look for enteric-coated capsules. The recommended dosages range from 400 to 600 milligrams for mild depression, up to 1,600 milligrams daily.

▲ Three times a day, take 300 milligrams of **St. John's wort**. In folk medicine, it was originally said to ward off witches. Now that witches are more or less a thing of the past,

Should I call **the doctor?**

A divorce, a death, a move, or a career change can give you temporary feelings of sadness, as you experience a loss or confront new challenges. Almost everyone experiences a mild depression at some point in life. But if your sadness lasts more than two weeks, or is accompanied by sleep and appetite changes (eating and sleeping too much or not at all), loss of interest in sex, and a reduced ability to concentrate, chances are you need treatment. Your doctor will be able to advise you whether you need psychotherapy, medication, or both.

more than 20 scientific studies have shown that St. John's wort can help ease mild depression, possibly by allowing certain brain chemicals to build up between nerve cells, as some antidepressants do. Opt for a brand standardized to 0.3% hypericin. Because this herb can cause sensitivity to sunlight, try to stay out of the sun as much as possible while you're taking it.

 5-HTP, which is one form of the amino acid tryptophan, is thought to work the same way Prozac does, by increasing serotonin levels. Take 100 micrograms 3 times a day of 5-HTP. But don't take this supplement for more than 3 months unless you have your doctor's consent.

 Take 1,000 milligrams three times a day of the amino acid **acetyl-L-carnitine**. It's chemically similar to acetylcholine, a neurotransmitter that acts in the muscles as well as the central nervous system. Acetyl-L-carnitine helps increase energy production in brain cells, protect nerve cell membranes, and improve both mood and memory.

 The mineral **chelated magnesium** is very important for restoring and maintaining healthy nerve function. Magnesium

Five Steps to Positive Thinking

Is your inner monologue bringing you down? Here's how to turn your thinking around:

1. Take a just-the-facts approach. Challenge irrational beliefs that chip away at your confidence. If you think everyone is laughing at you, demand evidence. Are they actually laughing? Could they be laughing at something else?

2. Don't be perfect. It isn't possible—but you knew that. So why worry if someone doesn't like you or you're not masterful and competent in every situation?

3. When something bad happens, don't automatically think the worst ("I failed the test because I'm stupid"). There are usually many reasons things go sour. Look at all of them objectively and focus on those you can change ("Next time, I'll do better if I study harder").

4. If self-examination does reveal a personal weakness, keep the implications from spiraling ("I can't do anything well"). And remember: Recognizing that you're weak in one area doesn't make you a weak person. Instead, it can help you identify where to invest more effort and guide you to your strengths.

5. Loosen your grip on the controls. Inevitably, things don't always go your way. Accept that the world isn't under your control and strive to be calm in the face of adversity. That way, two problems—the upsetting situation and your reaction to it—are whittled to just one.

is a key component in the production and function of sero-tonin. Supplements may help alleviate anxiety and depression. Follow the dosage recommendations on the label.

➤ Take one **vitamin B-complex** supplement each morning with food. Low levels of vitamin B have been linked with depression. Look for a brand with 50 micrograms of vitamin B_{12}, 400 milligrams of folic acid, and 50 milligrams of the other B vitamins.

The Power of Prevention

➤ **Get enough sleep**. Studies have shown that people who get less than eight hours of sleep, night after night, tend to have lower serotonin levels than those who get full nights of rest. To help ensure a good night's rest, try to go to bed at the same time every evening and rise at the same time every morning—even on weekends.

➤ **Shut off the TV**. Research suggests that the longer you watch television, the more your mood suffers. Watching hours of reruns, movie marathons, or game shows may seem like a way to relieve stress and fill up on entertainment. But studies have shown that, to the contrary, people who watch a lot of television usually have intensified feelings of isolation.

Diarrhea

When a case of the runs has you running to the bathroom, your aims are two: Stave off dehydration, and avoid anything that will make the diarrhea worse. If you can stay close to home, simply let the problem "run" its course (and don't forget to drink plenty of fluids). If you can't, try astringent teas, eat more soluble fiber (which soaks up excess fluids in the intestine), or try an ancient Chinese "cure."

What's wrong

Normally, as food goes through your digestive tract, the large intestine soaks up extra water. Sometimes, though, it doesn't, and you get rid of the fluid in your stool—a bothersome problem we call diarrhea. Common causes include viral infections, like flu; exposure to parasites or foreign versions of the bacterium *E. coli* while traveling; bacterial food poisoning; and intolerance to an ingredient in dairy foods. Diarrhea that lasts for days or weeks, however, can point to irritable bowel syndrome. And diarrhea that's not quickly resolved can cause dehydration, which is especially dangerous in infants and the elderly.

Tame Diarrhea with Tannins

↪ Drink **black tea** sweetened with **sugar**. The hot water helps with rehydration, and tea contains astringent tannins that help reduce intestinal inflammation and block the absorption of toxins by your intestines. The sugar improves sodium absorption.

↪ Tannin-rich **blackberries** have long been used as folk treatments for diarrhea. Make blackberry tea by boiling one or two tablespoons of blackberries or dried blackberry leaves in 1½ cups water for 10 minutes, then strain. Drink a cup several times a day. You can also purchase store-bought blackberry tea bags, but check that they contain blackberry leaves and not just blackberry flavoring. **Raspberry tea** is also said to be effective.

Root Out the Problem

↪ Capsules of dried **goldenseal**, made from the bright-yellow root of a perennial herb, appear to kill many of the bacteria, such as *E. coli*, that cause diarrhea. The key compound in the herb is berberine, which is so effective that goldenseal is sometimes called an "herbal antibiotic." Take two or three 125-milligram capsules daily until the diarrhea improves.

Infuse Your Body with Fluids

↪ When your diarrhea is considerable, you need to replace your body's supply of water and electrolytes, which include sodium, potassium, and chloride. These keep your heart beating properly and play many other crucial roles as well. Mix up the perfect **electrolyte drink** by stirring a half-teaspoon of salt and four teaspoons of sugar into a quart of water. Add a little bit of orange juice, lemon juice, or salt substitute for potassium. During the day, drink the full quart. Don't use more than this amount of sugar or salt; much more, and you're likely to become dehydrated.

➤ Brand-name sports drinks like **Gatorade** can also replace lost electrolytes.

➤ When you're caring for a child with diarrhea, use an oral rehydration solution such as **Pedialyte**, which is designed specifically to replace kids' electrolytes.

➤ If your diarrhea is mild and you're not dehydrated, just drink **flat sodas** (you don't want the carbonation to give you gas) to keep your fluid levels normal. Leave one soda open in the refrigerator for a few hours so it de-fizzes. Take sips for a few hours, then start drinking as much as you comfortably can until you're getting a pint of fluid each hour.

Rebuild Your Diet

➤ Start by eating only foods that are see-through, like **chicken broth** and **Jell-O**. Broth is an especially good choice, since it supplies your body with water as well as electrolytes from the salt. Stick with these "clear" foods for a day or two. But **avoid fruit juices**. They can contain large amounts of a kind of sugar called fructose, which many people have trouble digesting even when they're feeling well.

➤ Spoil yourself with the **BRAT diet**. BRAT stands for bananas, rice, applesauce, and toast. All are bland and soothing, and the bananas and applesauce contain pectin, a type of soluble fiber that soaks up excess fluid in your intestine and slows down the passage of stool. (Avoid apple juice, however, which can make diarrhea worse.)

➤ **Carrots** are another soothing source of pectin. Cook some carrots until they're soft, then drop them in a blender with a little water and puree into a baby-food consistency. Eat a quarter to a half-cup each hour.

➤ **Avoid** foods that are rich in **roughage**, which can be hard to digest. That means no beans, cabbage, or Brussels sprouts.

Should I call **the doctor?**

If your diarrhea lasts longer than two days, recurs frequently, or is accompanied by light-headedness, a fever, intense cramping, or blood or pus in the stool, call your doctor. A particularly serious form of diarrhea is related to *Clostridium difficile,* a bacterium that occurs normally in many children under the age of two and in some adults as well. When antibiotics are overused, *C. difficile* alters the flora in the intestine in such a way that it causes a particularly foul-smelling form of diarrhea. It requires immediate treatment.

Traveler's diarrhea, also known as Montezuma's revenge or turista, is the bane of international travelers, usually caused by exposure to foreign strains of bacteria in the food or water. Before you board the plane for points remote, learn how to avoid spending the bulk of your trip in the bathroom.

🖝 Take Pepto-Bismol before, during, and after the trip. A number of studies have shown that this can help prevent traveler's diarrhea. And even if the diarrhea has started, Pepto-Bismol can help reduce the severity of the symptoms. Following the directions on the package, chew two pills four times a day or (if you're taking the liquid) one tablespoon four times a day.

🖝 Before you leave, start taking acidophilus capsules twice a day to boost the number of beneficial bacteria in your intestine. Continue taking them while you're abroad. Follow the dosage instructions on the bottle. But make sure you're getting live bacteria. One brand is VSL3, produced by Probiotica.

🖝 Drink only water or drinks that are in sealed bottles or cans, or water that has been boiled for three to five minutes. Use bottled water to brush your teeth and cook, and never have ice cubes in your drinks (you don't know what water was used to make them).

🖝 Acidic drinks like orange juice and sodas are also good for diarrhea prevention because they help keep the bacterium *E. coli* in check.

🖝 Eat only cooked foods and fruits that you can peel yourself.

🖝 Have a glass of wine with meals. In the lab, wine has been shown to kill the bacteria that cause traveler's diarrhea. There's no research to say whether drinking wine actually helps, but if you enjoy wine (in moderation) anyway, why not? You're on vacation!

🖝 Eat **yogurt** containing **"live cultures"** as specified on the label. "Cultures" refers to beneficial bacteria like *Lactobacillus acidophilus* and *Bifidobacterium*. Eating yogurt with live cultures helps restore healthy levels of these bacteria to your intestine and may speed recovery from diarrhea. If your diarrhea is related to taking antibiotics, which kill good and bad bacteria indiscriminately, it's especially important to replenish the "good guys." If you don't like yogurt, buy **acidophilus pills** and follow the dosage instructions on the label.

Solve It with Psyllium

🖝 One good treatment for diarrhea is also a remedy for the opposite problem—constipation. Ground-up **psyllium seeds** soak up excess fluid in the intestine, making the stool bulkier. They are the key ingredient in Metamucil, Fiberall, Hydrocil, and other natural-fiber products. Take one to three tablespoons mixed in water each day.

Ancient Chinese Treatment

Here's an old Chinese remedy for diarrhea. We have no idea if it works, but it can't hurt. Peel and crush 2 cloves **garlic**, add 2 teaspoons **brown sugar**, boil in ¾ cup water, and drink 2 to 3 times a day. Because garlic has potent antibacterial properties, it may kill the bacteria behind many cases of diarrhea.

The Power of Prevention

If you find that you frequently get diarrhea after consuming milk and other dairy products, delete those foods from your diet. They contain a sugar called lactose, and some people are **lactose intolerant**. If you do eat dairy, take supplements (such as Lactaid) that contain the enzyme lactase. Or only eat low-lactose dairy, such as yogurt, aged cheddar, and Lactaid-brand milk.

Steer clear of any products containing the sweeteners **xylitol, sorbitol**, and **mannitol**. These are often found in diet candies and sugar-free gum, but also in strawberries, prunes, cherries, and peaches. Our bodies cannot easily digest the sweeteners.

Wash your hands with soap and warm water before you prepare foods and after you handle raw meats. And be sure to wash all plates and cooking implements that have come in contact with raw meat.

To prevent food poisoning, **defrost foods in your microwave or the refrigerator**, not on the counter.

Avoid taking large doses of **vitamin C**, which may give you diarrhea.

If you customarily take antacids that contain **magnesium hydroxide**—like Maalox or Mylanta—consider **switching to another brand**. This ingredient can cause diarrhea.

Skip it!

As soon as diarrhea hits, you might be tempted to swallow an over-the-counter anti-diarrhea medication. Don't—particularly during the first few hours. Diarrhea is a natural way for your body to quickly rid itself of bacteria and irritants, so you don't want to slow down this process.

Dry Mouth

If a lack of saliva makes it hard for you to lick envelopes or even talk, you'll definitely want to wet your whistle. First, talk with your doctor about what might be causing your kisser to be parched. Consider an over-the-counter saliva substitute such as Salivart, Xero-Lube, or Optimoist. Drinking plenty of plain old H_2O will keep your mouth moist, as will the other tricks in this chapter.

What's wrong

The mucous membranes in the mouth have become abnormally dry due to a lack of saliva. Dry mouth can be caused by medications or by the radiation, chemotherapy, and surgery that are used to treat oral cancer. And sometimes it's the result of an autoimmune condition called Sjögren's syndrome, in which the immune system attacks moisture-producing glands in the body. Dry mouth is also related to aging: About 40 percent of people over age 65 have it. Because saliva protects us from oral infections and tooth decay, having dry mouth can lead to bad breath, mouth sores, cavities, and fungal and bacterial infections in the mouth.

Check Your Medicine Cabinet

➤ Dozens of common medications can cause dry mouth. **Check the label** or package insert of any drug you're taking to see whether dry mouth is listed as a side effect. If it is, ask your doctor if you can switch to a different drug. Frequently implicated drugs include many antihistamines and decongestants as well as Prozac (fluoxetine), Norvasc (amlodipine), Paxil (paroxetine), and Vasotec (enalapril).

Just Add Water

➤ Carry a **water bottle** with you and sip water frequently. Swirl each sip around in your mouth before you swallow. You should be going through 64 ounces—half a gallon—each day.

➤ To stimulate saliva flow, squeeze in some **lime** or **lemon juice** or add one-half teaspoon **apple cider vinegar**.

Make Your Mouth Water

➤ Chew **sugarless gum** or suck on **sugarless hard candy** to stimulate the flow of saliva. Sugar-free gums with the ingredient xylitol can help reduce cavity-causing bacteria.

➤ Keep a **red-pepper** shaker handy at the table. The same "hot stuff" that makes your eyes water and your nose run can make your saliva pour forth. Add just a touch to spice up your meals.

➤ The herb **echinacea**, taken in tincture form, has been shown to help stimulate saliva production. Drink 10 to 15 drops of tincture in a glass of juice. This remedy is safe to use every hour, if needed, for up to eight weeks.

Avoid These Drought-Inducers

🍂 **Limit** your intake of **coffee** and other **caffeinated drinks**, as well as **alcohol**. These cause you to urinate more frequently, which makes your body lose more fluids.

🍂 **Eschew sodas**, even those without caffeine. If your mouth is dry, you don't have enough saliva to break down the acid they contain.

🍂 **Shun salty foods** or **highly acidic drinks** like orange juice and lemonade. These can cause pain if your mouth is too dry.

🍂 Keep **sugary snacks** to a minimum.

🍂 **Tobacco** dries up saliva. If you smoke, try to stop.

Add a Little Night Moisture

🍂 To avoid getting dried out at night, use a **humidifier** or **vaporizer** in your bedroom.

Swishing Well

🍂 If you use a store-bought mouthwash, pick one that **doesn't contain alcohol**, which dries your mouth and can irritate already-sensitive gum tissues.

🍂 For a homemade mouthwash, mix one-eighth teaspoon **salt** and one-quarter teaspoon **baking soda** in a cup of warm water. Rinse your mouth and spit. This solution will counteract acids in your mouth and rinse away infectious agents.

Teeth Treatments

🍂 Choose a toothpaste that **doesn't contain sodium lauryl sulfate (SLS),** which can irritate mouth tissues. Brands without SLS include Rembrandt's Natural and Biotene's Dry Mouth Toothpaste.

🍂 Make sure you **brush** and **floss** thoroughly. Saliva is important for clearing away food debris in your mouth, and when your mouth is dry, this food can stick around.

Keep Your Mouth Shut

🍂 When you inhale through your nose, you moisturize the air going into your body. But when your sinuses are clogged, you naturally do a lot of mouth breathing, and that means you're taking in a lot of dry air. Take steps to treat a **sinus condition or allergies,** and you will also help prevent dry mouth.

Should I call **the doctor?**

If you notice that your mouth is unusually dry for more than a few days, talk to your doctor or dentist. A consultation is especially important if the condition prevents you from eating or speaking normally or your mouth is red and irritated. When you discuss it with your doctor, be sure to mention any medications you're taking, since they may be contributing to the problem.

Earache

There's nothing like an earache to take you back to the less pleasant aspects of childhood. Put simply, earaches are no fun. You can approach the problem from the outside in, using carefully chosen eardrops or even a bit of garlic juice, or from the inside out, with soups and gargles that help drain mucus and expand the Eustachian tubes. Warm and cold treatments can also help you weather the pain.

What's wrong

Something has probably gone awry in the middle ear, which is the tiny space located behind your eardrum. A thin tunnel called the Eustachian tube runs from the middle ear to the back of the throat. That tube allows fluid to drain away, and it's also a passage where the pressure inside your ear adjusts to meet outside air pressure. The common cold virus can cause fluid to accumulate in the Eustachian tube, triggering significant pain. Bacteria thrive in the fluid, leading to middle-ear infections. These are all too common in children, but can strike adults as well. If you get an earache from flying, the cause is probably excessive air pressure rather than infection.

Just Drop In

Place 3 to 5 drops of 3% commercial grade **hydrogen peroxide** into the painful ear canal every 3 to 4 hours. This will help quell infection, inflammation, and pain.

Warm a bottle of **baby oil** or **mineral oil** under hot water for a minute, then drip a few drops of the warm oil into your ear to help ease discomfort.

Drain It, Dry It

Try a **spicy chicken-noodle soup** or fiery bowl of **chili**. The spiciness gets your mucus flowing and can help your ears drain, relieving painful pressure.

Gulp down plenty of **water** every day. The muscles that work when you swallow help your Eustachian tubes open up, allowing your ears to drain.

Gargle with warm **salt water**. It helps increase blood circulation to the Eustachian tubes and decreases swelling that may be blocking them.

Make a healing remedy of **echinacea** and **goldenseal**. Echinacea helps your body fight off the infection, and goldenseal helps dry out the fluid in the ear. Put a dropperful each of tincture in a quarter-cup of water, then drink the mixture every two to three hours. Or buy a tincture containing both herbs.

Use an **extra pillow** to prop your head up slightly more than normal while you're sleeping. This will help your ears drain, easing pressure.

Warm and Chill

👉 Lie on your side and place a comfortably warm **hot-water bottle** or **heating pad** over your ear. Or use a towel dampened with hot water. The soothing warmth increases circulation to the ear and also helps relieve pressure.

👉 Use a **hair dryer** as another source of warmth. Set the dryer on the lowest warm temperature, hold it at least six inches from your ear, and direct the airstream down your ear.

👉 To draw inflammation away from the affected ear, wear **ice-cold socks** on your feet and apply a **warm compress** to your ear. Saturate cotton socks in ice water, wring them out, and place them against the soles of your feet. Then pull wool socks over the cold socks to hold them in place. Simultaneously, place a hot moist compress over the painful ear.

Ease the Ache with Garlic

👉 Eat one or two raw cloves of **garlic** every day. The pungent bulb helps fight viruses and bacteria. Some brave souls just chew on the cloves. A more palatable alternative: Chop up the fresh garlic, mix it with olive oil, and spread it on your favorite bread.

👉 If you find that raw garlic tends to upset your stomach, take a capsule of **garlic supplement** with each meal.

👉 Squeeze a clove of garlic and put a few drops of the juice in your ear. Because garlic has antibacterial properties, this direct approach fights infection.

Turn on the A and C

👉 Take 50,000 IU of **vitamin A** twice a day until your symptoms improve. Vitamin A is an antioxidant that helps fight infection, promote healing, and maintain mucous membranes. If you still need to take it after a week, drop the dosage to 25,000 IU a day, and continue taking it for another week—but not longer unless you consult with your doctor.

👉 Take 1,000 milligrams of **vitamin C** and 500 milligrams of **flavonoids** three times a day until the infection is gone. Vitamin C is an antioxidant that promotes healing. When it's combined with flavonoids—anti-inflammatory components extracted from plants—the vitamin works even better.

Should I call **the doctor?**

See your doctor if your ear is extremely painful, if it hurts for more than a week, or is accompanied by 100°F fever or higher. You should also tell the doctor about any fluid discharge from your ear, feelings of dizziness, or painful sensations when you chew. Sudden, intense pain, followed by some relief, could indicate a ruptured eardrum. Other common signs of ruptured eardrum are discharge (sometimes with blood), muffled hearing, a ringing in the ears, and a feeling of dizziness or vertigo. If you have these symptoms, see your doctor before trying any of the remedies in this chapter.

The Power of Prevention

A few simple steps can keep you from having to worry about aching ears:

- When you have a cold, **blow your nose gently.** If you honk too forcefully, you can push bacteria back into your middle ear from your sinuses and trigger an infection.

- Frequent ear infections can be a sign of **food allergy.** Most often, the troublesome foods are dairy products, wheat, corn, peanuts, or oranges. Try removing these foods from your diet for several weeks to see if you feel any better. Then add them back one at a time. If your ears start aching, delete the food from your diet for good.

- Chew **sugarless gum** that contains the sweetener xylitol, which comes from birch trees and is also found in strawberries and plums. In one study, children who chewed two pieces of the gum five times a day for two months had 40 percent fewer ear infections. The xylitol may cut down the growth of bacteria that cause middle-ear infections. One brand of gum is VitaDent.

Earwax

Just the annoyingly resonant rumble of your own voice is probably enough to tell you that earwax buildup is out of hand. Easy-does-it earwax removal is usually a two-part project—first the insertion of something to soften up the wax, then an ear wash to flood the gunk and carry it out. Easier said than done? Here are some tips to help the wax wane.

Try an Ayurvedic Approach

🔊 Gently **massage** the area directly behind your earlobe to help loosen the wax. Then **tug the earlobe** while opening and closing your mouth.

Soften and Rinse

🔊 Fill an eyedropper with warm **hydrogen peroxide** that is body temperature or a little warmer. Lie down or tilt your head so that your blocked ear is pointing up. Drip the hydrogen peroxide into the ear until it feels full. Wait three minutes before tilting your head the other way over a washbasin or hand towel to let the peroxide drain out. Now tilt your head back once more and gently squirt warm water from a bulb syringe into your ear. Let it settle, and then tilt your head to the other side and let it run out again. Clean away the water and softened wax from your outer ear with a washcloth or cotton balls.

🔊 An alternative to the hydrogen peroxide treatment is using oil to soften the wax. Tilt your head and place a few drops of warm **baby oil** or **mineral oil** into the affected ear with an eyedropper. Let the oil work its way down into your ear. You can leave it in for up to one hour. Then, with a bulb syringe, squirt in some warm water to flush the oil out of your ear. Turn your head from side to side as long as the water continues to drain out.

What's **wrong**

Earwax, known medically as cerumen, is normally a useful substance. Secreted by glands in the outer portion of the ear canal, that wax traps dirt before it gets deep into your ears. When your ears produce too much wax, however, or you inadvertently push it into the canal by trying to clean it out, cerumen can form a hard plug deep in the ear. This can cause earaches, ringing in the ears, hearing loss, and balance problems.

Should I call **the doctor?**

Air Your Ear

After you finish washing the wax out of your ears, use a **hair dryer** to air-dry them. Set the hair dryer on its coolest setting and hold it about 12 inches away.

The Power of Prevention

Whenever you're washing up, rub a damp washcloth around the loops and whorls of your outer ear. **Never stick a cotton swab** or any other type of probe into your ear, however. You'll ram the wax deeper, and since there are no oil glands deep in the ear canal to keep the wax soft, it will harden like a rock. The other risk is that you could puncture your eardrum or scratch your ear canal.

Cut down on consumption of **saturated fats** found in animal foods like meat and dairy, and minimize your consumption of the hydrogenated fats found in commercially baked snacks and other processed foods. Some experts believe these types of fats prompt your body to produce greater amounts of earwax and also make the wax stickier. Replace these dietary fats with healthier ones, such as those found in cold-water fish, nuts, and seeds.

If you wear a **hearing aid**, wipe it with a tissue every night at bedtime when you remove it. This gets rid of wax residue before it has time to accumulate.

For people who have a lot of ear hair—particularly some older men—it helps to trim the hair with small scissors or a battery-operated **ear-hair trimmer.** The trimming will help prevent earwax from getting enmeshed in hair around the opening of the ear canal.

Eczema

Like so many skin problems, eczema can itch worse than a bad conscience. Your avenues of attack: Keep out of the water (that means no dishwashing, frequent hand washing, or long showers) as much as possible. Guard your skin with a thick, heavy-duty cream—not a watery lotion. Stay away from eczema aggravators, such as harsh soaps and anything you discover you're sensitive to. And, hard as it may be, avoid scratching.

Rash Relief

To cool your itch, soak a washcloth in ice-cold **milk** and lay the cloth onto the itchy area. Repeat several times daily as needed.

For an oozing rash, apply **calamine lotion**. It can help with the itching and also dry out the rash.

Soak and Seal

Add **colloidal oatmeal** to your bath. This ground oatmeal floats suspended in the water and is soothing to itchy skin. A well-known brand is Aveeno.

Keep your baths and showers under 10 minutes. In fact, **don't bathe every day** if you don't have to. Eczema tends to get worse when skin is dry, and excessive bathing washes away the protective oils that keep your skin moist.

Use **lukewarm water** in the tub or shower instead of piping hot water.

After you bathe, use a **heavy cream-based moisturizer** to guard the skin against irritants. Even petroleum jelly or solid vegetable shortening, such as Crisco, works well. Avoid water-based lotions, as well as lotions that contain fragrance.

Get Some Internal Revenue

Eat more foods rich in essential fatty acids like omega-3s, which help reduce inflammation and allergic reactions. You'll find these in rich amounts in **walnuts, avocados, salmon, mackerel,** and **tuna.**

What's wrong

There are several types of eczema. Atopic eczema, the most common, usually occurs in people with a family history of allergies or asthma. Symptoms— red, itchy skin—generally begin before the age of five, then reappear periodically during adulthood. During acute flare-ups, the skin may be marked with small, fluid-filled blisters. Over time, excessive scratching causes patches of skin to look thick and scaly. Skin damaged by eczema and scratching is prone to bacterial infections. Another type of eczema, called contact dermatitis, stems from contact with an irritating substance such as detergent, soap, and cosmetics.

Should I call the doctor?

If your eczema is widespread or keeps recurring despite your self-care treatments, contact your doctor. And you'll need a doctor's attention as soon as possible if an itchy patch of skin begins to show signs of infection. These include crusting sores, pus, red streaks on the skin, excessive pain, swelling, or fever.

🍂 Another good source of omega-3s is **flaxseed oil.** Take up to one tablespoon each day; it won't hold up in high cooking temperatures, so drizzle it on salad, mix with yogurt, or hide it in other foods.

🍂 Take 400 IU of **vitamin E** each day to help counteract itchy, dry skin. (*Off-limits* . . . if you're taking blood-thinning drugs unless you have your doctor's approval.)

🍂 Take 25,000 IU of **vitamin A** each day for up to 10 days when you're having an eczema flare-up, then reduce the dose to 10,000 IU daily. But check with your doctor first. Long-term use of vitamin A can result in osteoporosis, and an overdose of this vitamin can cause thickening and peeling of skin and hair loss.

🍂 **Zinc** helps your skin heal, and it also helps your body make use of essential fatty acids. Take 30 milligrams of zinc daily. Because zinc can interfere with copper absorption, also take 2 milligrams of copper each day if you continue to take zinc for more than a month.

Go to Gotu

🍂 The herb **gotu kola**, used externally, can help ease itchy skin conditions. Look for a commercial cream or extract. If you use the extract, dilute it first (5 parts water to 1 part extract). Alternatively, you can make a cup of the tea, soak a cloth in it, and use the cloth as a compress. To make the tea, steep 1 teaspoon of the dried herb in 1 cup of hot water. Steep for 10 minutes, then strain.

🍂 As an alternative to gotu kola, look for a cream containing **chamomile, licorice,** or **witch hazel.** All of them reduce skin inflammation.

Stop the Scratching

🍂 If the itchy spot is somewhere way too accessible, such as your wrist or the back of your hand, **cover it with a small bandage** to remind yourself not to scratch.

🍂 Some people scratch in their sleep. If you're waking up with scratched skin, **wear thin cotton gloves** (or, in a pinch, a pair of socks) over your hands at night.

🍂 **Keep your fingernails cut short** to minimize skin damage if you do scratch.

Strong Medicine

In December 2000, more than 40 years after the last new drug was developed to treat eczema, a prescription ointment called tacrolimus (brand name Protopic) was approved by the FDA. In studies, more than two-thirds of the people who used the ointment showed improvement, many after using the ointment for only one week. If you have eczema that isn't helped by home remedies, see a dermatologist about a prescription for this new medicine.

The Power of Prevention

◆ Many experts feel that **food allergies** play a significant role in eczema, particularly in children under the age of two. In kids, the problems most often come from eggs, dairy, peanuts, soy, wheat, and tree nuts. In adults, the troublesome foods are usually dairy, wheat, eggs, yeast, and citrus products. Eliminate all these foods from the diet for about a month, then bring back one at a time for three days to see if the skin reacts. In children, this food–elimination diet may produce a visible change in a short time. Dramatic change is rarer in adults, but still, you might note some improvement.

◆ During winter months, use a **humidifier** in your bedroom to help keep your skin moist.

◆ To minimize sweating in the summer, which can aggravate eczema, run the **air conditioner.**

◆ Rely on your **dishwasher** as much as possible to avoid contact with detergents and water.

◆ When you do wash dishes, wear a pair of **lined rubber gloves** or wear rubber gloves over a pair of thin cotton gloves. **Avoid direct contact with latex**, since it can cause allergic reactions—and make eczema worse—in some people.

◆ Keep your use of laundry chemicals to a minimum. Use a **fragrance-free** and **dye-free** detergent. **Avoid bleach, fabric softeners**, and **dryer sheets.**

◆ Give your clothes an **extra rinse** in the washing machine to remove all traces of detergent.

◆ Consider whether something you've touched has caused a breakout, and steer clear of these substances in the future. **Contact dermatitis** can be caused by nickel used in earrings and other jewelry, as well as latex, cosmetics, perfumes, and cleaning agents.

Skip it!

Over-the-counter corticosteroid creams, like hydrocortisone, can help tame eczema. But if you use them too often—say, every day for more than three weeks—they can thin and damage the skin.

Eyestrain

Your eyes may be the windows to your soul, but when overworked, they become doorways to pain, headaches, and blurred vision. Unfortunately, eyestrain is all too common when people spend countless hours staring into the glare of computer monitors and televisions. What to do about it? Give the eyes as much rest as possible. And make some adjustments to your computer and your work habits to make life easier on the eyes.

What's wrong

Hold a dumbbell in your outstretched hand, and your muscles soon grow tired. The same happens to eyes when you overtax them. If the eye muscles that focus your vision don't have a chance to relax, you'll soon feel the strain. You may even have trouble focusing. And if you're squinting in bright sunlight, a case of eye ache comes on very quickly.

Rest 'Em, Blink 'Em, Close 'Em

Whenever you're working on a task that requires close concentration, **take a break** every 20 minutes or so. Look at a faraway object—a picture on the opposite wall, or a view out the window—for at least 30 seconds. By allowing your eyes to shift focus, you give them a rest.

Try to **blink often**—every few seconds or so—when you're paying close attention to your television or computer screen. Blinking moistens your eyeballs and relaxes your eye muscles.

If you have a long task that involves prolonged staring, **close your eyes** periodically. Even if you just shut your eyelids for a few seconds, you'll get some immediate relief.

Warm and Cool Relief

Another way to **relax your eye muscles**: Briskly rub your hands together until they grow warm, and gently place the heels of your palms over your closed eyes. Hold them there for a few seconds.

If you soak a washcloth or hand towel in **cool water**, wring it out, and lay it over your eyes for five minutes, it will relieve strain.

Cool your eyes with sliced **cucumber.** Lie on your back and place one slice over each closed eye. Leave on the slices for two or three minutes, or replace the first pair with another, cooler set of slices.

Glasses for Your Neck

If you wear bifocals, you can get neck strain from working at a computer. That's because with bifocals, the "reading" lens is at the bottom of the glasses, so you have to tilt back your head to see the computer screen.

Ask your eye doctor to prescribe another pair of glasses that will give you clear vision at a distance of 20 inches, so you can read what's on the monitor without awkward head tilting.

Tear Up

↖ For eyestrain that is related to dry eyes, use **artificial tears**, available at pharmacies. Two common brands are Viva-Drops and Similasan.

Adjust Your Monitor

↖ **Turn the contrast** on your computer monitor to high. Letters and images become crisper.

↖ Adjust your **chair height** so you're looking slightly downward at the screen. Tilt the screen to meet your gaze.

↖ Make sure that your eyes are at least **20 inches** from the screen.

↖ Adjust your computer screen or close the shades near your work area so that you **don't have window-glare** on the screen.

↖ If glare still bothers you, attach a special **antiglare filter** to the screen.

↖ **Clean the dust** off the screen regularly to improve clarity.

↖ If you're mildly nearsighted, try reading or viewing the computer screen **without your "distance" glasses.** Your eyes might be more comfortable that way.

↖ Choose a **bigger font** so your eyes don't have to work as hard to focus, or use the **zoom feature** to enlarge what you're viewing.

Use Shades

↖ In any bright sun—even in the winter—**wear sunglasses.** They will reduce eyestrain that comes from squinting. Choose sunglasses with yellow, amber, orange, or brown lenses. Light in the blue part of the spectrum is what makes us squint, and these lenses block it.

Should I call
the doctor?

If your eyes frequently feel strained and home remedies don't work, if your vision grows increasingly worse, or you're very sensitive to light, consult an eye doctor. Also, if dizziness or double vision occurs suddenly and doesn't go away when you rest your eyes, be sure to talk to your doctor promptly.

Light Up Your Life

~ When you're reading, be sure the light is adequate so you don't have to strain to see the print. The best results are with a **gooseneck lamp** directed so that the light falls on the page. Generally, a lower-watt bulb in a gooseneck lamp is more effective than a higher-watt bulb in a shade lamp. A 45- to 65-watt indoor floodlight bulb should give plenty of illumination.

~ Don't settle for one reading lamp in an otherwise dark room. Be sure that **other lights are also turned on.** If there's too much contrast between the light where you're reading and the rest of the room, your pupils will constantly have to narrow and widen to adjust for the difference.

~ **Avoid** reading or working under **fluorescent lights.** They may flicker, contributing to eyestrain. The incandescent light from ordinary lightbulbs is your best bet.

Check Out Cheap Specs

~ After age 40 or so, many people have trouble focusing on nearby objects—a condition called presbyopia. If your distance vision is still fine and both eyes are focusing equally, try purchasing an inexpensive pair of **reading glasses** from your local drugstore to resolve the problem.

Fever

If your forehead is fiery with fever, you could reach for acetaminophen (Tylenol) or ibuprofen (Advil) to lower your temperature. (Don't treat fevers with aspirin in anyone under the age of 19; doing so can trigger a potentially fatal disease called Reye's syndrome.) But if your fever is 101°F or below, don't be afraid to let it run its course; Mother Nature has raised your temperature for a reason. If you're uncomfortable, though, and you want to take action, try these tips to tame the fires within.

Be Cool

❧ Take a **bath in lukewarm water.** This temperature will feel plenty cool when you have a fever, and the bath should help bring your body temperature down. Don't try to bring a fever down rapidly by plunging yourself into cold water; that tactic sends blood rushing to internal organs, which is how your body defends itself from cold. Your interior actually warms up instead of cooling down.

❧ Give yourself a **sponge bath.** Sponging high-heat areas like your armpits and groin with cool water can help reduce your temperature as the water evaporates.

❧ When you're not bathing, place **cold, damp washcloths** on your forehead and the back of your neck.

Sweat It Out

❧ Brew a cup of **yarrow tea.** This herb opens your pores and triggers the sweating that is said to move a fever toward its end. Steep a tablespoon of herb in a cup of freshly boiled water for 10 minutes. Let cool. Drink a cup or two until you start to sweat.

❧ Another herb, **elderflower**, also helps you sweat. And it happens to be good for other problems associated with flu and colds, like overproduction of mucus. To make elderflower tea, mix two teaspoons of the herb in a cup of boiled water and let it steep for 15 minutes. Strain out the elderflower. Drink three times a day as long as the fever continues.

What's **wrong**

A fever is often a sign that your body is fighting off infection. As your white blood cells battle with microscopic invaders, they release chemicals that raise your body temperature, making the environment less friendly to viruses and bacteria. A fever in adults is generally regarded as a temperature higher than 100°F. In infants and young children, any fever should be treated. But in older children and adults, a fever of 101°F or below doesn't necessarily need to be treated unless the person has intense discomfort because of sweating, chills, or both.

Should I call **the doctor?**

Contact your doctor if you have a temperature of 103°F or higher, if a temperature of 101°F lasts longer than 72 hours, or if your pulse is above 110 beats per minute. Also, call your doctor immediately if the fever is accompanied by a stiff neck, a severe headache, extreme drowsiness, shortness of breath, burning with urination, red streaks near a wound, a severe rash, or sensitivity to light. Any fever in infants younger than six months should be brought to the attention of your pediatrician right away.

Old **wives' tale**

Forget the old saying about "starving a fever" to make it go away. (Actually, the original saying was "feed a cold, *stave* a fever," *stave* meaning to prevent.) Fasting will weaken you just as you should be preserving your strength. Even if you don't feel like eating, at least have some chicken soup and toast or other soothing foods.

~ Drink a cup of hot **ginger tea**, which also induces sweating. To make the tea, steep a half-teaspoon minced gingerroot in 1 cup just-boiled water. Strain, then drink.

Fight Fire with Fire

~ Sprinkle **cayenne pepper** on your foods when you have a fever. One of its main components is capsaicin, the alarmingly hot ingredient that's found in hot peppers. Cayenne makes you sweat and also promotes rapid blood circulation.

Soak Your Socks

~ Try the **wet-sock treatment**, a popular folk remedy for fever. First warm your feet in hot water. Then soak a thin pair of cotton socks in cold water, wring them out, and slip them on just before going to bed. Put a pair of dry wool socks over the wet ones. This approach helps ease a fever by drawing blood to the feet, which dramatically increases blood circulation.

~ Another way to draw blood to the feet is with a **mustard footbath.** In a basin large enough for your feet, add two teaspoons of mustard powder to two pints of hot water, then soak.

Get Between the Sheets

~ An old folk remedy for treating a fever is to **soak a sheet in cold water** and wrap yourself in it. Today, doctors advise against lowering your body temperature too quickly, so if you try this remedy, use slightly cool, not cold, water. Cover the wet sheet with a large beach towel or blanket, then lie down for about 15 minutes. Unwrap yourself when the wet sheet starts to get warm.

Fill Up on Fluids

~ When you have a fever, it's easy to become dehydrated. Drink 8 to 12 glasses of **water** a day or enough to make your urine pale. A sports drink like Gatorade can also be helpful. It not only replaces fluids lost to dehydration but lost minerals as well.

~ Orange juice and other fruit juices rich in **vitamin C** are good choices, since the vitamin C assists your immune system in fighting off infection.

~ Cold **grapes** provide hydration—and a soothing treat.

Flatulence

Just bringing up the subject of flatulence starts people giggling, but when it's you who's passing gas, you probably don't regard it as a laughing matter. Instead of worrying about running to another room to avoid embarrassment, take the wind out of your sails by cutting out gas-causing foods, chewing on gas-relieving seeds after a meal, and taking steps to help your body digest food more completely.

Deflate Your Diet

⌁ Certain foods are notorious for producing gas. Avoid them if they give you trouble. They include **beans, cabbage, bran, cauliflower, broccoli, onions, prunes, raisins,** and **Brussels sprouts.** Also on the list are eggs, which have some sulfur in the yolk that contributes to odorous gas.

⌁ Take preventive measures before you eat. A product called **Beano,** which you can add to beans and other troublesome foods, supplies enzymes you need to digest these foods without gas. Take the Beano tablets or droplets at the start of a meal, following the label for dosage directions.

⌁ Before you cook beans, **soak them overnight.** The next day, pour off the old water, then replenish with fresh water for boiling. This will remove some of the carbohydrates that cause gas.

⌁ **Avoid** candies and gums that contain the sweeteners **sorbitol, xylitol,** and **mannitol.** Your body has trouble digesting them, and when they get to your colon, the resident bacteria there feed on them and produce gas.

⌁ **Cut down on fructose,** a sugar found in honey, fruits, and fruit juices. Like other sweeteners that are difficult to digest, fructose stays in the colon, where bacteria feed on it and create gas-rich fermentation. Don't cut out whole fruit from your diet, but go easy on fruit juice and honey if they bother you.

⌁ If you're adding more **fiber** to your diet, do it gradually. Fiber is terrific for your health, but adding a lot to your diet all at once can lead to an odoriferous end.

What's **wrong**

The average adult passes gas between fifteen and twenty times a day. Typically, this is just the release of air we've swallowed or gases—including carbon dioxide, methane, and sulfur dioxide—produced while we're digesting food. Such gases are the odorous by-products of hungry bacteria that linger in the digestive tract, feeding off partially digested carbohydrates. If you're constipated, you might have excessive flatulence because you're not expelling gas during regular bowel movements. Also, people who can't properly digest dairy foods—a problem dubbed lactose intolerance—often have problems with flatulence.

Should I call **the doctor?**

If flatulence bothers you continually, and is accompanied by diarrhea and bloating, talk to your doctor. He or she may want to examine you for other indications of the condition known as irritable bowel syndrome. Also, severe flatulence that doesn't go away can sometimes be a symptom of gallbladder problems, an inflammatory condition in the intestines, or colon cancer.

Look to Lactaid

If you are lactose intolerant, take a supplemental over-the-counter product such as **Lactaid** when you consume milk, cheese, ice cream, or other dairy foods. Or look for **reduced-lactose milk** at the supermarket. People who have trouble digesting dairy lack an adequate supply of the enzyme lactase, which breaks down lactose, the sugar in milk. Since the body's lactase supply often dwindles as we grow older, you may develop this problem in later years, even if it hasn't been an issue before.

Not sure if you're lactose intolerant? Trying **giving up dairy foods** for a few days and see if it makes a difference.

After-Your-Meal Medicine

If you've eaten a big meal that is likely to make you flatulent, drink a cup of **ginger tea.** It stimulates digestion so food won't linger in your intestines, contributing to gas. To make the tea, steep a quarter-teaspoon of powdered ginger in a cup of hot water for five minutes.

Peppermint also helps minimize gas and improve digestion. Drop dried peppermint leaves into a cup of freshly boiled water, and steep for 5 to 10 minutes. Strain and drink. You can use this remedy three or four times daily as needed. (*Off-limits* . . . if you have gastroesophageal reflux or heartburn.)

Fennel seeds, which have a pleasing licorice scent, have been used for hundreds—perhaps thousands—of years to reduce gas and improve digestion. Chew half a teaspoon of the seeds after a meal, or sprinkle them on your food. You can also make fennel tea by steeping 1 to 2 teaspoons crushed dried seeds in 1 cup just-boiled water for 10 to 15 minutes. Strain, then drink. Caraway seeds have a similar effect.

Give gas the **papaya** treatment. Papaya contains an enzyme called papain that helps the body break down food. Buy papain tablets, or juice half a papaya, add an equal amount of water, and drink.

Lavender is said to be effective against gas. It can also help soothe after-meal cramps in the stomach and intestines. To make a tea, steep 1 or 2 heaping teaspoons of lavender flowers and steep for 10 minutes in a cup of boiling water, then strain and drink.

Act with Acidophilus

Take an **acidophilus** supplement each day for two to four weeks. Acidophilus is one of the "friendly" bacteria that inhabit the large intestine and keep gas-causing bacteria in check. Follow the dosage directions on the label. Or eat yogurt that contains live cultures (check the label).

Curl Up for Comfort

If you're feeling painful abdominal cramps, try to find a private place where you can **lie down** for a few minutes. Lying on your back, pull your knees up toward your chest. This posture allows the gas to escape more easily, relieving discomfort.

Get on the Move

Walking is a particularly good way to encourage gas dispersal. In hospitals, it's the first thing that doctors recommend to postoperative patients to help them get bowels working again. Stroll a few blocks and see if it helps.

The Power of Prevention

To reduce the swallowed air that goes into your stomach, **avoid** drinking through **straws.**

Don't chew gum. When you do, you automatically swallow more air.

Avoid carbonated sodas and other bubbly drinks, which carry gas into your digestive tract.

Chew food thoroughly. When you gulp it down, you swallow more air. Also, large chunks of food take longer to digest, which means they linger in the digestive tract, where feeding bacteria launch the fermentation process.

Did you **know?**

You're more likely to feel gassy on an airplane. In a plane, the air pressure around you is lower than usual—about what you'd find if you were 8,000 feet high in the mountains. Due to simple physics, when the pressure around you falls, the gas inside you expands.

Skip it!

Over-the-counter antigas medications containing simethicone break large gas bubbles into smaller bubbles. But that bubble breakdown doesn't fix flatulence. You'll still have gas. And products that contain activated charcoal, which allegedly soaks up gas, haven't been proven to do so.

Foot Odor

Do people turn up their noses when you slip off your shoes? Has the family dog fallen in love with your footwear? There are plenty of solutions that go way beyond baking soda to stop the sweat, eat the odor, and keep your feet from smelling like... smelly feet. In particular, many people swear by using an antiperspirant on their tootsies.

What's wrong

Your feet are the natural habitat of millions of bacteria, which thrive on your sweat and skin cells. By-products produced by these bacteria are what give feet that stinky smell. When you seal your feet in a pair of shoes and they pour out sweat, you give the bacteria more food to feast on. Foot odor can also be caused by poorly controlled fungal infections, such as athlete's foot. People with diabetes or heart disease, as well as elderly people in general, are often more apt to develop foot infections and foot odor due to less-than-adequate circulation.

Give Feet the Underarm Treatment

It shouldn't come as a surprise that the same **antiperspirant** you use on your underarms can also keep feet less sweaty (and therefore less smelly). Simply spray or roll it on before putting on your shoes and socks.

Wash your feet daily in warm water using a **deodorant soap** or **antibacterial soap**.

Turn Up the Heat

Especially if you are prone to athlete's foot or nail fungus, blow-dry your feet with a **hair dryer** that's turned to the lowest temperature. This helps avoid infection and reduces moisture.

Soak 'Em and Scent 'Em

Try a **black tea footbath.** Boil two tea bags in a pint of water for 15 minutes. Remove the bags and dilute the tea with two quarts of water. Let the mixture cool down if necessary, then soak your feet for 30 minutes. Repeat daily. The tannic acid in strong black tea kills bacteria and closes pores to help your feet sweat less.

Make an odor-fighting foot soak by adding a cup of **vinegar** to a basin of warm water. For more odor-fighting force, add a few drops of **thyme oil.** The oil contains a strong antiseptic that kills odor-causing bacteria. Soak your feet for 15 to 20 minutes a day for a week. (*Off-limits* . . . if you have any open sores or broken skin.)

If you don't have access to thyme oil, you can easily buy a product that contains it: **Listerine.** Try adding a splash to your footbath. (The same cautions as with thyme oil apply.)

Fragrant Foot Rub

Lavender oil not only smells good, it helps kill bacteria. Rub a few drops onto your feet and massage it in before you go to bed at night. Cover your feet with socks. Before trying this remedy, check to make sure the oil won't irritate your skin by putting one drop on a small area.

Salt Your Dogs

Mix two cups of **Epsom salt** into one to two gallons of warm water in a bucket or basin. Soak your feet for 15 minutes twice a day. The Epsom salt acts as an astringent to reduce sweating, and may kill bacteria.

Try an Acne Treatment

Apply **benzoyl peroxide** 5% or 10% gel to the bottoms of your feet to fight bacteria. Why not? It works on your face.

Powder Power

Dust your feet with **talcum powder** or **foot powder** before you put on your shoes and socks. It will absorb odor-causing sweat.

Two other good foot powders to try are **baking soda,** which neutralizes odor, and **cornstarch,** which absorbs moisture.

Dress Well for a Better Smell

Change your socks at least once a day, replacing them with a clean pair.

Alternate between at least **two pairs of shoes.** After you've worn one pair, set them aside and let them air out for at least 24 hours.

Wear shoes with **open-mesh** sides or sandals that allow your feet to "breathe." Your feet will also breathe better if you wear **cotton socks** rather than polyester.

Should I call **the doctor?**

If these remedies don't fix your foot odor, consult your doctor or a podiatrist. You may have an infection that requires an antibiotic or a prescription antifungal medication.

Treat Shoes with Savvy

❧ Check the care instructions on your athletic shoes. If they're washable, toss them into the **washing machine** at least once a month.

❧ Store your shoes in a place that's **bright** and **ventilated**—not in a dark closet, where bacteria thrive.

❧ Each time you put your shoes away, insert a sachet filled with cedar chips into them. You can also try products that consist of mesh pouches filled with **zeolite.** Zeolite is a natural volcanic mineral that attracts odors and traps them. Expose the reusable pouch to the sun for six hours to discharge the collected odors.

❧ Buy odor-absorbing **insoles** and cut them to fit. Replace them every three to six months.

❧ If your shoes have removable insoles, **take them out to dry** every time you remove your shoes. And toss them in the washer from time to time.

Gout

The agony of gout can start very quickly. One minute, you're skipping along with a smile on your face and a song in your heart. The next, you're in excruciating pain. Your first instinct might be to reach for aspirin—a wrong move. Aspirin slows the excretion of uric acid, which only makes things worse. A better bet is naproxen (such as Aleve or Naprosyn) or the prescription drug indomethacin (Indocin). Then you can turn to these home remedies to further reduce pain. Pay special attention to drinking plenty of water to dissolve the uric acid crystals.

Lift Off and Ice Down

 ﹀ During an acute attack, try to **stay off your feet** as much as possible and keep the affected joint elevated. This probably won't be a problem. When gout is at its worst, most people can't even bear the weight of a bed sheet on the painful joint.

 ﹀ If you can stand to, apply an **ice pack** for 20 minutes or so. The cold will dull the pain and bring down the swelling. Wrap the ice in a cloth to protect your skin. Use the ice pack 3 times a day for two or three days.

Try the Cherry Remedy

 ﹀ **Cherries** are an old folk remedy for gout. They contain compounds that help neutralize uric acid. Cherries are also a source of anti-inflammatory compounds. So if you feel an attack of gout coming on, try eating a handful or two of cherries right away. If they aren't in season, buy canned cherries or black cherry juice (drink 1 to 2 cups; try mixing it with pineapple juice).

 ﹀ Alternatively, you can take **cherry fruit extract pills**, which are available at health-food stores. The recommended dose is 1,000 milligrams once a day (for maintenance) or three times a day (for attacks).

 ﹀ Don't like cherries? Some people swear by **strawberries** for gout.

What's **wrong**

When too much uric acid (produced in the liver and excreted in the urine) builds up in your system, needle-sharp crystals of the compound can form in the fluid that cushions your joints. You may feel like you have shards of glass jammed into your joints. This painful inflammatory condition, known as gout, usually occurs in men over age 40 (it takes years for uric acid crystals to build up). Though it most often affects the big toe, gout can strike the wrist, knee, elbow, or another joint. Besides pain, gout can cause severe swelling.

Should I call **the doctor?**

Anytime you develop a tender, swollen joint, call the doctor, even if you've had similar attacks in the past. Gout can mimic other conditions, such as joint infection, so the doctor should first confirm a diagnosis by drawing liquid from the affected joint and examining it under a microscope to confirm the presence of uric acid crystals. Prescription drugs for gout are available. But before you take one, make sure your doctor knows about every medication and supplement you're already taking, since some of those may be increasing your risk of gout.

Pill Power to the Rescue

➤ Daily doses of **fish oil** or **flaxseed oil** can ease the inflammation in the joints. These oils are rich sources of a potent anti-inflammatory agent known as eicosapentaenoic acid (EPA). The typical dosage of fish or flaxseed oil is 1,500 milligrams a day (about a tablespoon).

➤ Another way to ease inflammation is with pills containing **bromelain**, an enzyme found in pineapple. The typical dosage for acute gout attacks is 500 milligrams three times a day between meals.

➤ Tablets containing **celery seed extract** seem to help eliminate uric acid. The typical dosage is two to four tablets a day.

➤ Long advocated by herbalists to treat joint inflammation, **nettle** also helps lower uric acid levels. Experts typically recommend 300 to 600 milligrams of a freeze-dried extract a day. Don't use nettle for more than three months at a time. (*Off-limits* . . . nettle in tincture form. Tinctures contain alcohol, which aggravates gout.) Another way to use nettle is to soak a clean cloth in a tea brewed from the leaves of nettle and apply it to the tender joint. If you pick this common weed yourself, wear gloves, long pants, and long sleeves to guard against nettle's stinging leaves.

Live on Water, Not Beer

➤ Drink lots of **water**—at least eight 8-ounce glasses a day. Fluids will help flush excess uric acid from your system. As a bonus, the water may help discourage kidney stones, which disproportionately affect people with gout.

➤ **Avoid alcohol.** It seems to increase uric acid production and inhibit its excretion. Beer is particularly bad—it contains more purines (see below) than other alcoholic beverages.

The Anti-Gout Diet

High-protein foods, as well as foods that contain chemical compounds known as purines, can raise levels of uric acid in the body. If you have gout, the list of foods to avoid includes meat-based gravy, organ meats like kidneys and sweetbreads, mussels, sardines, liver, herring, fried foods, refined carbohydrates (such as white flour), oatmeal, yeast-containing foods like beer and baked goods, asparagus, peas and beans, spinach, and cauliflower.

To Tame the Pain, Mind Your Meds

~ If you're taking a diuretic—for high blood pressure, for instance—ask your doctor about **alternatives.** Diuretics eliminate excess fluids from the body; as a side effect, they reduce the amount of uric acid that passes in the urine. Less passes, more stays, and the worse your gout.

~ Gout can also be **triggered by niacin,** or **nicotinic acid,** which is often prescribed for high cholesterol. If your doctor has prescribed niacin for you, ask about alternatives.

Fast Not, Hurt Not

~ Losing weight can help keep gout at bay, but going on a crash diet or fasting is a big mistake. Drastic dieting causes cells to release more uric acid. If you're overweight, **lose weight slowly** and sensibly—two pounds a week at most.

Did you **know?**

Because only the better-off could afford foods like herring, shrimp, and fatty meats, known to trigger gout attacks, gout was once known as rich man's disease.

Gum Problems

If you're hurting and you want relief right now, you can walk into any drugstore and buy a tube of gel containing the topical anesthetic benzocaine. Or try a gargle or a soothing gum massage as described below. But your real war is with plaque. Control the plaque with regular visits to the dentist and dedicated brushing (use a soft-bristled brush and pay special attention to your gum line) and flossing and you should be able to give gum problems the brush-off.

What's wrong

Are your gums puffy? Do they bleed when you brush? You probably have gingivitis, a form of gum inflammation caused by plaque, a sticky film of food particles and bacteria that accumulates on your teeth. Plaque is irritating to your gums. If it isn't removed by brushing and flossing, it can turn into hard mineral deposits that are even more irritating (and which can be removed only by a dentist). Left untreated, gingivitis eventually leads to full-blown gum disease, in which the gums pull away from the teeth. The resulting germ-filled pockets can lead to painful abscesses and chronic bad breath, and can even cause your teeth to loosen and fall out.

Play by the Numb-ers

➤ To soothe gum pain and reduce swelling, swish for 30 seconds with **salt water** (one teaspoon mixed into a glass of warm water).

➤ Alternatively, rinse your mouth with **hydrogen peroxide** diluted 50:50 with warm water. Like salt, hydrogen peroxide dulls the pain and helps kill bacteria.

➤ Place a wet **tea bag** against the painful area. Tea contains tannic acid, a powerful astringent that shrinks swollen tissues and helps stanch bleeding. Think of it as a styptic pencil for your gums. If bleeding and inflammation persist, fold the bag in half and bite down on it.

➤ Apply an **ice pack** (wrapped in a cloth) to your cheek near the painful area. Ice helps reduce swelling, and the cold acts as a local anesthetic.

➤ Dab your gums with a paste made of **baking soda** and water. Baking soda kills germs and helps neutralize the acids they secrete. Don't go overboard, though; too much baking soda can damage tender gum tissue.

Rub for Relief

➤ What do you do for sore muscles? **Massage** them! And your gums benefit from massage too. Just grip them between your thumb and index finger, and give a series of gentle squeezes. That helps boost circulation to painful, irritated tissue, helping gums heal faster.

To enhance the soothing effect of a gum massage, try doing what practitioners of Ayurvedic medicine recommend: Massage your gums with **coconut oil.**

Another way to massage your gums is with a soft wooden **dental stimulator**, which you can pick up at any drugstore. Insert it between two teeth, point the tip so it's at a 45-degree angle to the gum line, circle gently for a few seconds, then move on to the next two teeth.

Buy a **Water-Pik** or another "oral irrigator," and use water pressure to clean and massage your teeth and gums where your toothbrush cannot reach.

A time-tested wound healer, **calendula** may help sore gums by reducing inflammation. Simply rub the tincture directly onto the gums.

Rinse and Gargle

Twice a day, gargle with a mouth rinse containing the B vitamin **folic acid.** Studies have shown that swishing twice a day with an over-the-counter folic acid solution helps with bleeding gums.

Rinsing your mouth with **chamomile tea** is said to be highly effective against gingivitis. Simply pour a cup of hot water over 3 teaspoons of the herb, steep for 10 minutes, then strain and cool. Mix up a large quantity and store it in the refrigerator.

Store-bought mouthwash can also help heal your gums. Choose a brand that contains **cetylpyridinium chloride** or **domiphen bromide.** These ingredients have shown significant plaque-reducing ability.

Should I call **the dentist?**

As long as you're having your teeth professionally cleaned and examined twice a year (more often if plaque formation is a problem), minor gum irritation does not require a visit to the dentist. Just consider your irritated gums a wake-up call that you need to pay more attention to brushing and flossing. Do call your dentist if you notice a change in the appearance of your gums, or if they start bleeding. For intense pain, schedule an immediate appointment, especially if you have fever and a swelling in the neck. You could have an abscess that needs prompt treatment.

Headaches

Oh, my aching head! In a world of traffic jams, tight schedules, and high-speed everything, it's no wonder we find ourselves popping an occasional pain reliever. For a bad headache, choose one that contains a combination of aspirin, acetaminophen, and caffeine. (*Off-limits*... if you have a bleeding disorder, asthma, ulcers, or liver or kidney damage.) But painkillers are only part of the solution. There's much more you can do to escape the thump and wallop of a throbbing noggin.

What's wrong

Specialists have identified a few major types of headache. Tension headaches seem to be caused by muscle contractions in the head and neck, and they're characterized by dull, steady pressure. Migraines originate with constriction and expansion of blood vessels in the head. There may be throbbing pain on one or both sides of the head, often accompanied by nausea and sensitivity to light or sound. Agonizing cluster headaches are sometimes triggered by drinking or smoking, and they come episodically in groups, or "clusters," followed by periods of remission.

Give It Some Good Press

With a firm, circular motion, **massage** the web of skin between the base of your thumb and your forefinger. Continue massaging for several minutes, then switch hands and repeat until the pain resolves. Acupressure experts call this fleshy area trigger point LIG4 and maintain that it is linked to areas of the brain where headaches originate.

Heat Up and Cool Down

Believe it or not, soaking your feet in **hot water** will help your head feel better. By drawing blood to your feet, the hot-water footbath will ease pressure on the blood vessels in your head. For a really bad headache, add a bit of hot mustard powder to the water.

For a tension headache, place a **hot compress** on your forehead or the back on your neck. The heat will help relax knotted-up muscles in this area.

It might sound contradictory, but you can follow up the heat treatment (or substitute it) by applying a **cold compress** to your forehead. (Put a couple of ice cubes in a washcloth or use a bag of frozen vegetables.) Cold constricts blood vessels, and when they shrink, they stop pressing on sensitive nerves. Since headache pain sometimes originates in nerves in back of your neck, try moving the compress to the muscles at the base of your skull.

Here's an alternative to a cold compress: Soak your hands in **ice water** for as long as you can stand it. While your hands are submerged, repeatedly open and close your fists. This works on the same principle as an ice pack on your head—the cold narrows your dilated blood vessels.

Try the Caffeine Cure

Have a cup of **strong coffee.** Caffeine reduces blood-vessel swelling, and thus can help relieve a headache. This is why caffeine is an ingredient in some extra-strength pain-killers like Excedrin. However, if you are already a heavy coffee drinker, skip this. Caffeine withdrawal can cause headaches, creating a vicious cycle.

Do Something Constrictive

Tie a **bandanna, scarf**, or **necktie** around your forehead, then tighten it just to the point where you can feel pressure all around your head. By reducing the flow of blood to your scalp, this can help relieve the pain caused by swollen blood vessels. You might try soaking the bandanna in vinegar, a traditional headache remedy.

Soothe with Scent

Certain essential oils—especially **lavender**—can help ease tension and relieve the pain of a headache. Gently massage a bit of lavender oil onto your forehead and temples, then lie back and enjoy the relaxing scent. For maximum relief, slip away to a room that's cool, dark, and quiet. The longer you can lie there quietly breathing in the aroma, the better.

In addition to lavender oil—or instead of it—use **peppermint oil.** The menthol it contains can help dissolve away a headache. Its fragrance at first stimulates, then relaxes, the nerves that cause headache pain.

If you have a vaporizer, add 7 drops **lavender oil** and 3 drops **peppermint oil**, then breathe in the relief. If you don't, try sprinkling a few drops of peppermint oil on a tissue. Inhale deeply several times.

Try wringing out two wet **peppermint tea bags** and place them on your closed eyelids or forehead for five minutes.

Should I call **the doctor?**

An occasional headache is usually nothing to worry about. But sudden, severe pain suggests a serious condition. Get immediate help if you develop an excruciating headache accompanied by blurry vision, or if you suddenly have difficulty moving any part of your body. Ditto if you get fever, a stiff neck, or if you have slurred speech or confusion, especially if you've received a blow to the head. Though it's not an emergency, you should talk to a doctor if you have three or more headaches a week or if you find yourself taking pain relievers on a daily or almost daily basis.

Did you **know?**

Frequent use of aspirin or ibuprofen can cause "rebound headaches" that start as soon as a dose begins to wear off. Solution: Quit the drugs cold turkey, even if it hurts.

Swallow Some Throb Stoppers

🍃 An anti-inflammatory, **ginger** was traditionally used to treat headaches, and it seems to work. Grind up a half-teaspoon ginger, stir it into a glass of water, and drink this "ginger juice." Or pour 1 cup hot water over 1 teaspoon freshly ground ginger, let the tea cool a bit, then drink it. Ginger is especially effective against migraines, though how it works is not well understood. Doctors do know that ginger has an effect on prostaglandins, hormonelike substances that

Migraines

Migraines are characterized by throbbing, excruciating pain, usually on one side of the head. Nausea, vomiting, sensitivity to light, or visual disturbances may accompany the pain. Doctors aren't sure what causes migraines, but they suspect an association with abnormal constriction and dilation of the arteries that supply blood to the brain. The problem tends to run in families. There are many possible triggers, including sensitivities to foods or food additives, stress, hormonal fluctuations during the menstrual cycle, oral contraceptives, caffeine withdrawal, changes in the weather or season, bright lights, and odors. Migraines are more common in women than in men.

It's easier to prevent a migraine than it is to treat one. Try these techniques:

🍃 An herbal remedy from Europe called Petadolex can help relieve and prevent migraines. Take one gelcap three times daily.

🍃 Avoid foods that contain lots of the amino acid tyramine. So-called trigger foods include cured and processed meats, such as bologna, hot dogs, pepperoni and sausage, aged cheeses, nuts and peanuts. Chocolate and red wine are other sources of tyramine.

🍃 The herb feverfew has the power to reduce the intensity and frequency of migraines. Follow the dosage recommendations on the label. You'll need to take the capsules every day—possibly for several months—to maximize the herb's preventive power.

🍃 Flaxseed oil is rich in essential fatty acids, which help your body produce fewer inflammation-causing prostaglandins, hormonelike chemicals that can constrict blood vessels. Take 1 to 2 tablespoons a day. Buy the cold-pressed oil, and keep it in the refrigerator to protect it from light and heat. Good-quality flaxseed oil has a pleasant, nutty flavor; sneak it into a smoothie or add it to a salad.

🍃 Although experts aren't exactly sure how, the B vitamin riboflavin can help prevent migraines. Doctors recommend starting at a daily dose of 200 milligrams, but some people need to take up to 400 milligrams daily before they get results.

🍃 A magnesium supplement may also help. In some studies, people reported that their symptoms were much improved by taking 200 milligrams of magnesium each day. If that doesn't work, you can take up to 600 milligrams daily.

🍃 At the first sign of a migraine, take one-third teaspoon of fresh or powdered ginger. Danish researchers discovered that ginger can help prevent the onset of migraines by blocking prostaglandins.

contribute to inflammation. Ginger also helps control the nausea that so often accompanies migraines.

🍃 Try drinking a cup of **rosemary tea**; some people say it helps keep a headache from getting worse. Pour 1 cup boiling water over 1 teaspoon of the dried herb, steep for 10 minutes, strain, and drink.

🍃 At least one grandmother counted on strong **black tea** with a few bruised whole **cloves** added. Tea contains caffeine, and cloves have anti-inflammatory properties, so the brew might indeed help a headache.

🍃 Down a large glass of **water** and see if it helps. Dehydration can cause a headache.

The Power of Prevention

🍃 If you grind your teeth or clench your jaw—either when you're awake or asleep—take steps to prevent the problem. You might need to wear a **mouth guard** at night. (See Teeth Grinding, page 225, for advice.)

🍃 **Eat at regular intervals.** There's evidence that a drop in blood sugar—the result of going too long without eating—can set the stage for headaches.

🍃 At least three days a week, spend 30 minutes walking, cycling, swimming, or doing some other form of **aerobic exercise.** These exercises are great stress-relievers.

Heartburn

Heartburn is definitely punishment, but it's not always clear why you've been sentenced. Some say, "Don't eat so much" or "Don't eat so fast." Others like to blame spicy foods like fiery Szechuan or acidic foods like grapefruit and oranges. As a first line of defense, visit the pharmacy for over-the-counter antacids like Mylanta or Maalox, or acid suppressors like Zantac and Pepcid AC. But the long-term goal is to pinpoint—and avoid—your all-too-personal heartburn triggers.

What's wrong

When stomach acid backs up into your esophagus, you feel a burning pain. What causes acid backups? A trapdoor of muscular tissue called the lower esophageal sphincter (LES) usually keeps stomach acid where it belongs. With heartburn, it allows acid to leak upward, a problem known as reflux. Large meals as well as certain foods can lead to heartburn. You're more likely to have heartburn if you're pregnant, overweight, or a smoker, or if you have a condition called hiatal hernia. Some medications, including aspirin, certain antibiotics, and some antidepressants and sedatives, may aggravate heartburn.

Douse the Flames

As soon as you feel the telltale flicker of heartburn, drink an eight-ounce glass of **water.** It will wash the acid back down your esophagus into your stomach.

To make a heartburn-easing tea, add 1 teaspoon of freshly grated **gingerroot** to 1 cup of boiling water, steep for 10 minutes, and drink. Long used to quell the nausea caused by motion sickness, ginger also helps to relax the muscles that line the walls of the esophagus, so stomach acid doesn't get pushed upward.

A tea made from **anise, caraway,** or **fennel seed** can also ease the burn, according to herbalists. Add 2 teaspoons of any of them to 1 cup of boiling water, steep for 10 minutes, strain, and drink.

Practitioners of Ayurvedic medicine, the traditional medicine of India, prescribe teas made of crushed **cinnamon** or **cardamom** to cool the heat of heartburn. Add 1 teaspoon of either crushed or powdered herb to 1 cup boiling water, steep, strain, and drink.

Don a Protective Coat

Marshmallow root is one of the oldest remedies known for heartburn. It produces a gooey, starchy substance called mucilage, which coats and protects the mucous membranes of your esophagus—just what you need when you feel like it's on fire. Stir 1 teaspoon powdered marshmallow root into 1 cup water and sip it. Drink three or four cups a day.

♦ You can make a similar soothing drink from **slippery elm.** Add one teaspoon of the powder to a cup of hot water, and drink a few cups throughout the day.

♦ A form of **licorice** called DGL also provides soothing mucilage. Take two or three chewable wafers three times daily on an empty stomach.

Put It in Neutral

♦ Saliva helps neutralize stomach acid. So chew a piece of **sugarless gum,** suck on a candy, or daydream about juicy steaks or buttery lobster—whatever it takes to get you to generate and swallow extra saliva.

♦ **Baking soda** is alkaline, so it neutralizes stomach acid. Mix a half-teaspoon baking soda and a few drops of **lemon juice** in a half-cup warm water. Don't drink the baking soda by itself. You need the lemon juice to dispel some of the gas baking soda creates in the stomach when it comes in contact with stomach acid—there have been cases where baking soda produced such a rapid internal reaction that it ruptured the stomach.

♦ The juices of vegetables like **carrots, cucumbers, radishes,** or **beets** help to tame the acid in the stomach due to their alkaline nature. Feel free to add a pinch of salt and pepper for flavor. If juicing vegetables is inconvenient or strange to you, just eat some raw vegetables.

The Power of Prevention

♦ No matter how terrible you feel, **stay upright.** Gravity is a powerful force, and if you're standing, the earth's pull helps keep acid in your stomach. Avoid bending over after a meal, and definitely don't lie down.

♦ If nighttime heartburn plagues you, eat meals at least **2 to 3 hours** before you turn in. The added time will give acid levels a chance to decrease before you lie down.

♦ You might also **elevate the head of your bed** four to six inches with large wooden blocks. When you're tilted at an angle while sleeping, gravity helps keep acid in the stomach.

Should I call **the doctor?**

An occasional episode of heartburn isn't serious. But frequent bouts may be one symptom of a viral infection. Recurrent heartburn could also be a sign of gastroesophageal reflux disease (GERD), which can cause or contribute to ulcers of the esophagus, chronic cough, dental problems, and even asthma and pneumonia. See your doctor if you get heartburn three or four times a week for weeks on end, if you wheeze or become hoarse, find it difficult to swallow, or lose weight rapidly. Finally, the symptoms of severe heartburn are often similar to those of a heart attack. If they arrive after a meal and are quelled by water or antacids, it's probably heartburn. But if you have a feeling of fullness, tightness, or dull pressure or pain in the center of the chest (possibly spreading to the shoulders, neck, or arms), shortness of breath, and/or light-headedness accompanied by a cold sweat, get immediate medical help.

Dodge These Edibles

"Food, glorious food!" rejoiced the hero of the musical *Oliver!* But if you're prone to heartburn, it's better to avoid certain foods—and drinks as well. Limit your consumption of the following:

Beer and wine, especially red wine. They tend to relax the LES, that important port of entry between your stomach and lower esophagus.

Milk. The fats, proteins, and calcium it contains can stimulate the stomach to secrete acid.

Coffee, tea, and cola. These caffeinated beverages also relax the LES, and they can irritate an already-inflamed esophagus.

Chocolate. It's loaded with two heartburn triggers—fat and caffeine.

Soda. The carbonation it contains can expand your stomach, which has the same effect on the LES as overeating.

Fried and fatty foods. They tend to sit in the stomach for a long time, where they can get that acid a-churnin'.

Tomatoes and citrus fruits and juices. They are acidic.

Peppermint and spearmint. They relax the LES.

Try **sleeping on your left side.** When you lie on your left side, the stomach hangs down and fluids pool along the greater curvature, away from the LES. Pooled fluids stay farther away from the esophagus.

Eat **smaller, more frequent meals** to minimize the production of stomach acid. And avoid eating too much in one sitting; doing so can force open the lower esophageal sphincter (LES), the thick ring of muscle that separates the stomach from the esophagus and keeps stomach acid where it belongs.

If you haven't done so already, **give up cigarettes.** Research shows that smoking relaxes the LES.

Hemorrhoids

Probably the only things more irritating than the burning, itching, and bleeding of hemorrhoids are the television commercials promising miraculous relief from them. Drugstore shelves are lined with products that help—creams, pads, ointments, and suppositories. As a rule of thumb, doctors say you should avoid OTC products that have ingredients ending in "caine." These have an anesthetic that provides immediate relief, but if used regularly, causes increased irritation. In addition to testing out OTCs, however, there are plenty of household remedies you'll want to try.

Fair Warming

↪ Fill the bathtub with 4 to 5 inches of **warm water**, then ease yourself into it. You should be in a seated position, but with your knees raised, allowing maximum exposure of the anal area to the warm water. You'll find that this eases the pain. What you can't feel is how the warm water encourages increased blood flow, and that, in turn, helps to shrink swollen veins.

↪ When you're using this "sitz bath," you can throw in a handful of **Epsom salt** before you plunge in to help constrict the hemorrhoids. Stir the water well to dissolve the salt.

↪ Rather than fill up a whole tub every time you want relief, you can purchase a **"sitz bath" basin** at most pharmacies and medical supply stores. Filling a small basin goes a lot faster than filling a whole tub, and since it's more convenient, you'll probably use it more often.

↪ For external hemorrhoids, apply a warm, wet **tea bag.** You can do it while sitting on the toilet. The warmth is soothing, and you get added benefit from one of tea's main components, tannic acid. It helps reduce pain and swelling, and since it also promotes blood clotting, this treatment helps stop the bleeding.

Saddle Up on Ice

↪ Fill a sturdy plastic bag with **ice**, wrap the bag in a thin cloth, and sit on it. The cold shrinks the swollen vessels,

What's **wrong**

Hemorrhoids are swollen veins in or around the anus that cause pain, itching, and, occasionally, bleeding. Internal hemorrhoids, the most common type, develop inside the anus. You might have some bleeding, but no pain. External hemorrhoids are the painful ones, and they, too, can cause some bleeding. Either kind may turn into a prolapsed hemorrhoid, a soft lump that protrudes from the anus. Prolonged sitting, pregnancy, and aging all contribute to hemorrhoids. If you frequently have constipation and strain when you're having a bowel movement, you can create hemorrhoids or make them worse.

Should I call **the doctor?**

Hemorrhoids don't require immediate medical attention. If you see bright red blood in the stool—a telltale sign—you first can try some self-treatment. But inflammatory bowel disease or a bowel infection can cause hemorrhoid-like symptoms. So if you see very dark blood or the stool looks black, call your doctor right away, as this is often a sign of intestinal bleeding. Also see your doctor immediately if you have significant rectal bleeding, persistent fecal incontinence, or the pain suddenly intensifies.

Did you **know?**

Hippocrates, the famous Greek physician who lived more than 2,400 years ago, knew that hemorrhoids were dilated anal veins. He recommended burning them away with a red-hot iron.

providing enormous relief. Sit in the chilly saddle for about 20 minutes. There's no limit on how often you can do this, but give yourself at least a 10-minute break between applications.

Do Dab, Don't Scratch

➤ Soak a cotton ball with undistilled **witch hazel** and apply to the hemorrhoids. It's rich in tannins, which cause the blood vessels to contract. Witch hazel is the main ingredient in the hemorrhoid pads Tucks.

➤ A dab of **Vaseline**, also contained in many over-the-counter hemorrhoid treatments, can help soothe the area.

➤ Liquid **vitamin E** and **wheat-germ oil** are both reputed to be effective. Put them on a cotton ball and apply it a few times a day.

➤ If you can find it in a natural foods store, try a salve containing **comfrey** or **marigold** to soothe and promote healing.

➤ Crazy as it sounds, a poultice made from **grated potato** is astringent and soothing.

Lounge Around

➤ A couple of times a day, find a comfortable couch, stretch out, and **put your legs up.** What's good for your frayed nerves is also good for your hemorrhoids. In this supine posture, you take the weight off your overstressed anal area. At the same time, you improve circulation to the roundabout that needs it. It's ideal if you can get 30-minute breaks for this assignment.

Go with the Grain

➤ Get more roughage into your diet. Research shows that **a high-fiber diet** can significantly reduce hemorrhoid symptoms, including pain and bleeding. Foods that are rich in fiber include whole-grain breads and cereals, fresh fruits and vegetables, brown rice, and nuts.

➤ When you're getting more fiber, you need to stay well hydrated to prevent constipation. Be sure to **drink enough fluids** so that your urine is pale, not dark, yellow.

Throne Room Policy

➤ Excuse yourself and **head for the bathroom whenever you have to go.** The trouble with waiting is that it leads to constipation. And that, of course, means you have to strain more when you go. And that invites hemorrhoids.

🖎 After a bowel movement, wipe with **plain, white, unscented toilet paper** that's been dampened under running water. Scented, colored toilet paper may have some aesthetic attractions, but any additional chemical can be an irritant.

🖎 After the initial clean-up, use facial tissues coated with an **unscented moisturizing cream.**

Limit Sitting and Lifting

🖎 Anyone who does a lot of sitting needs to do some standing as well. If you're tied to your desk most of the time, take a **five-minute walk** every hour or so. Every time you get up, you ease the rectal pressure that leads to hemorrhoids.

🖎 Heavy lifting puts pressure on the anal area. If there's a couch or dresser that needs lifting, claim a bad back and **ask for volunteers.**

🖎 If you usually lift weights when you work out, make sure you **skip the squat thrusts.** Every time you crouch down, then lift up again, you put direct pressure on your rectum. Also avoid any exercise that involves sitting for long periods, such as cycling on a stationary bicycle.

Tried...

Vicks VapoRub is a little-known home remedy for hemorrhoids.

...and true

There's no harm in trying this, putting it on the outside of the anus. People say it doesn't sting—but you'll have to try it for yourself to find out.

High Blood Pressure

Three out of ten people who have high blood pressure don't know they have it. Of those who do know, about seven out of every ten people don't have their blood pressure under control. So if you have no idea what your blood pressure is, ask your doctor to check it. If you've already been diagnosed with hypertension, be sure to follow the advice your doctor has given you. The cornerstones of treatment are exercise and diet changes. Even if your doctor has prescribed pressure-lowering medication, these lifestyle efforts are essential.

What's wrong

A high blood pressure reading means your heart is working harder than it should to pump blood, and your arteries are stressed. That's risky. If you don't lower your blood pressure, you'll face an increased risk for stroke, heart attack, kidney disease, and other deadly illnesses. You are considered to have high blood pressure (hypertension) when systolic pressure (the top number) is 140 or higher or the diastolic pressure (bottom number) is 90 or higher. But whenever your blood pressure readings start to creep upward, your doctor will urge you to take measures to control it.

Make a DASH for It

DASH is short for Dietary Approaches to Stop Hypertension, and in studies, this special diet has proved remarkably effective at lowering blood pressure. The gist of the diet is this: It's **low in saturated fat, cholesterol,** and **total fat**, with an emphasis on **fruits, vegetables, whole grains,** and **low-fat dairy foods.** The DASH diet can produce positive results in as little as two weeks. For a free copy of the diet, write to the National Heart, Lung, and Blood Institute Health Information Center, Box 30105, Bethesda, Maryland, 28204-0105, or download a copy at www.nhlbi.nih.gov/health/public/heart/hbp/dash/.

Ease up on the salt shaker. Eating too much salt causes your body to retain water. The effect is the same as adding more liquid to an overfilled water balloon: Pressure rises. In a follow-up to the DASH study, researchers found that the biggest drop in blood pressure came when people followed the DASH diet and also limited themselves to 1,500 milligrams of sodium a day. That's less than a teaspoon of salt a day.

Even if you don't add salt to your food at the stove or the dinner table, you may still be getting loads of "hidden" salt in packaged and processed foods, especially snacks, meat products, and canned soups. So before buying foods, **read labels carefully** to find out the sodium content. Look for low-salt soups and crackers, and rinse canned beans before using them.

Other Dietary Do's and Don'ts

⤳ Even if you don't follow the exact guidelines of the DASH diet, you'll see major benefits if you just make sure you eat lots of **fresh fruits** and **vegetables.** Vegetables can be raw or cooked. The point is to get five servings a day. You also want five daily servings of fruits—dried, fresh, frozen, or canned. Fruits and veggies are important sources of potassium, magnesium, and fiber—all of which help keep your arteries healthy.

⤳ **Oatmeal** has a special ability to lower blood pressure as well as cholesterol levels, as repeated studies have shown. Its beneficial effect seems to come from a form of soluble fiber known as beta-glucan. Start every day with a bowl of oatmeal, and you'll most likely see your pressure drop.

⤳ **Cut back on alcohol.** Heavy drinkers tend to have high blood pressure. If you do drink, limit yourself to one drink a day if you're a woman, two a day if you're a man. One drink is 12 ounces beer (regular or light), 5 ounces wine, or 1½ ounces 80-proof liquor (like whiskey).

Liberate Some Extra Pounds

⤳ Carrying extra weight forces the heart to pump harder. That's why blood pressure rises as body weight increases. If you're overweight, **losing as little as 10 pounds** can lead to a significant reduction in blood pressure.

Stamp Out Those Cigarettes

⤳ **If you smoke, quit.** Compounds in tobacco smoke contribute to hardening of the arteries by causing injury to blood vessels. And the nicotine in cigarettes causes blood vessels to constrict. That's bad for anyone, but it's especially bad for people who have high blood pressure.

Should I call **the doctor?**

If you've been diagnosed with high blood pressure, call your doctor immediately if you experience chronic headache, heart palpitations, shortness of breath, fatigue, nosebleeds, blurred vision, flushed face, frequent urination, or ringing in the ears. These symptoms suggest that your blood pressure is not being adequately controlled.

Is That Blasted Honking to Blame?

We all know that driving in heavy traffic can increase our stress levels. Now a study from Germany suggests that just the sound of traffic can send blood pressure soaring. The study of 1,700 people, conducted at the Robert Koch Institute in Berlin, found that people who live in areas of heavy traffic were twice as likely to be getting treatment for high blood pressure as were people residing on quiet streets. People who kept their windows open at night, in spite of the racket, were at highest risk.

At-Home Pressure Checks

Some people get so nervous when a doctor checks their blood pressure that they experience a temporary rise in blood pressure. If you're one of them, you can get a more accurate picture of your blood pressure by buying a blood pressure monitor and taking your own readings at home. The most reliable monitors have an inflatable arm cuff and a stethoscope, but the latest generation of automatic blood pressure monitors are quite accurate as well (and easier to use). Once you get the hang of it, you can take a reading any time of the day or night. By averaging out the readings, you'll get a true picture of your pressure.

Shake a Leg

 At least three times a week—and preferably five—get 30 minutes of **brisk exercise.** This advice might seem off the mark, since most kinds of exercise temporarily *raise* blood pressure. But when you work out regularly, you help keep your resting blood pressure at a safe level. Running, brisk walking, bike riding, and swimming are excellent choices.

Seek Peace

 Consider **getting a pet.** Whether it's cuddling a puppy or gazing at a tankful of colorful fish, interacting with animals has been shown to bring marked decreases in blood pressure.

 Watch the way you speak. Studies suggest that loud, fast talking goes hand in hand with high blood pressure. Practice **speaking in a lower tone** (and at a slower pace), even when you're upset or angry.

 Learn to meditate. This isn't New Age silliness. Research shows that meditation really does affect blood pressure, apparently by lowering levels of stress hormones in your body. To begin, choose a simple word or phrase to focus on. Close your eyes and relax all your muscles. Breathing slowly and naturally, repeat your word or phrase every time you exhale. As you do this, try to assume a passive attitude. Don't try to evaluate whether you're relaxed or "doing well"—just concentrate on your words and your breathing. Do this once or twice a day for 10 to 20 minutes.

 Engrossing **hobbies** such as gardening or sculpting may be just as good as meditation.

Supplement Your Efforts

🍃 Take 350 milligrams a day of **magnesium.** The mineral helps relax the smooth muscle tissue that lines blood vessels, allowing them to open wide. Magnesium is especially effective at lowering high blood pressure associated with pregnancy, but consult your doctor before taking any supplement when you're pregnant. Look for a magnesium supplement in the form of magnesium orotate or magnesium glycinate.

🍃 Take 100 to 300 milligrams of a standardized **hawthorn** extract a day. Hawthorn has long been known to dilate arteries. It seems to work by interfering with an enzyme that constricts blood vessels. That enzyme is angiotensin-converting enzyme (ACE), the same enzyme that some blood pressure drugs target. If you currently take medication for high blood pressure, consult your doctor before taking this herb. Hawthorn may take several weeks or even months to build up in your system and have an effect.

🍃 **Garlic** helps lower blood pressure, too, although it's not known why. Some experts recommend simply eating one clove of raw garlic a day. Others say to take four to six 600-milligram capsules or tablets a day, in divided doses. Choose enteric-coated capsules for best results.

🍃 Take **fish-oil supplements** to boost your intake of omega-3 fatty acids. These "good" fats come from cold-water fish like mackerel and salmon, and a typical supplement contains 1,000 milligrams. Taking three or four doses a day can help to reduce high blood pressure. Omega-3 fatty acids inhibit the body's production of substances, such as prostaglandins, that narrow the arteries.

High Cholesterol

The top three places you're likely to find unwanted sludge are in your plumbing pipes, in the fuel lines of your car, and in your arteries. The first will stop your sink, the second your travel, and the third your life. To keep your arteries from getting gummed up—or to clean them out if they're already in trouble—you'll need to lower your LDL level, and also try to boost your HDL level. For every 1 percent drop in your total cholesterol, your chances of having a heart attack fall by 2 to 3 percent. And for every 1 percent increase in your HDL, your risk drops by about 3 percent.

What's wrong

Inside your arteries, a dangerous change has taken place in the balance of fatty substances that circulate in your bloodstream. There is too much of the "bad" type of cholesterol, called low-density lipoproteins (LDLs). This is the type that gums up your arteries and raises your risk for heart attack and stroke. Meanwhile, you probably don't have enough "good" cholesterol, known as high-density lipoproteins (HDLs). These are the molecules that act as "garbage trucks," carrying LDL away to the liver for disposal.

Factor Out the "Bad" Fats

Eliminate as much **saturated fat** as possible from your diet. That means switching to leaner cuts of meats and lower-fat versions of dairy products such as milk, ice cream, cheese, and yogurt. Cut out ground beef altogether.

Run screaming from **palm oil** and **coconut oil**, which are very high in saturated fat. These so-called tropical oils are found in some processed foods.

Another type of fat, called trans fat, or **trans-fatty acids**, may be just as bad for your arteries as saturated fat. Store-bought cakes, doughnuts, cookies, chips, and other snack foods are often loaded with these fats, which are created when hydrogen is added to vegetable oils. To find them, look for the word "hydrogenated" on the package's nutrition label. In the United States, manufacturers have been required to list trans fats on package labels since 2006.

Eat more fresh fruits, vegetables, and **whole grains.** That's the easiest way to feel full as you cut back on meat and other fatty foods. In addition to being low in fat and cholesterol-free, plant foods contain lots of cholesterol-lowering fiber and heart-healthy vitamins and antioxidants.

Meat lovers should consider **bison, ostrich,** and **venison.** These game meats have a fraction of the fat found in grain-fed beef (the kind in most supermarkets). In fact, they are as low-fat as most fish. Marinate them to improve their tenderness.

Get More Good Fats

~ Numerous studies have shown that **olive oil** not only lowers LDL but also raises HDL. One study found that people who ate about 2 tablespoons of olive oil a day had lower LDL levels in just one week. Use it in garlic bread, salad dressings, in place of margarine, and in place of other oils when sautéing.

~ Enjoy **nuts.** They are packed with heart-healthy unsaturated fats, including omega-3s. Walnuts and almonds seem to be especially good at lowering LDL. Eat a shotglass-size serving a day and watch your numbers drop. But nuts contain a lot of calories, so make sure you eat them instead of—not in addition to—other snacks.

~ Have an **avocado** a day and you might lower your LDL by as much as 17 percent. True, avocados are very high in fat, but it's mainly the unsaturated kind.

~ Eat **peanut butter!** That's right, peanut butter. Yes, it's high in calories, but most of the fat it contains is unsaturated. Buy a "natural" brand that contains no hydrogenated oils.

Fish for Omega-3s

~ **Fish** is much more than a replacement for meat. It contains omega-3 fatty acids, which actually lower LDL cholesterol. Aim to eat fish three times a week—even if it's canned tuna. Your best bets are mackerel, tuna, and salmon, all very high in omega-3s. Sardines are great sources too.

~ If you absolutely won't eat fish, take a daily **fish-oil supplement** that contains both EPA and DHA (two types of omega-3 fatty acids). Take 1,000 milligrams twice a day.

~ Like **clams?** Indulge! Clams are high in sterols, chemicals that prevent your body from absorbing cholesterol.

~ **Flaxseeds** are great sources of omega-3 fats. Grind them and add to your yogurt or cereal. One study found that eating 2 tablespoons of flaxseed daily cut LDL cholesterol by 18 percent. You can also use flaxseed oil in salad dressing.

Eat Your Oatmeal

~ **Oatmeal** is a rich source of soluble fiber, which forms a kind of gel in your intestine to reduce your body's absorption of the fat you eat. Eating 1½ cups a day could lower your LDL

Should I call **the doctor?**

Your doctor should keep track of your cholesterol levels through regular screening tests. Ask your doctor for a copy of the report that breaks out LDL and HDL cholesterol so you'll know what your levels are. (The report will probably list other cardiovascular risk factors as well, such as total cholesterol and triglycerides.) If your cholesterol is high, your doctor may prescribe a cholesterol-lowering drug called a statin. But you'll still want to improve your diet, lose weight, and get more exercise.

12 to 24 percent. Choose quick-cooking or old-fashioned oats over instant oatmeal.

    ◣ Other especially good sources of soluble fiber include **prunes, barley, beans (legumes), eggplant**, and **okra.**

    ◣ Not getting enough soluble fiber in your diet? Try **psyllium**, found in dietary fiber supplements like Metamucil, Fiberall, and Hydrocil Instant. Research shows that taking about 10 grams a day for eight weeks can reduce LDL by 7 percent.

Put the Squeeze on Cholesterol

    ◣ Fresh-squeezed or straight out of the carton, **orange juice** can lower cholesterol. Participants in a recent study increased their HDL levels 21 percent and lowered their LDL/HDL ratio 16 percent by drinking three glasses a day for a month.

Why Not Wine?

    ◣ **Alcohol**—no matter what kind you drink—**raises HDL levels.** "Moderate" means one drink a day for a woman, and two a day for a man. If you drink more than that, the damage could outweigh any benefits. Red wine offers additional benefits: powerful antioxidants that come from the grape skin.

Get into the Sporting Life

    ◣ Lace up your **walking shoes**, and move along briskly for 30 minutes each day. Or climb on a Stairmaster and log your 30 minutes in the temperature-controlled climate of a health club. Or join the Y and get your laps in after work. The benefits of **regular exercise** are incontrovertible. Studies show that physical activity will improve the ratio of HDLs to

Niacin: Should You or Shouldn't You?

At high doses, the B vitamin niacin can lower cholesterol. But don't take it unless your doctor recommends a particular dose and monitors your health while you're taking it. Niacin does have the effect of lowering LDLs while raising HDLs—and in this respect, it resembles prescription medications. However, the amount of niacin you need to reap these benefits is very high, and when you take excessive doses, you risk many potential side effects. Some people get uncomfortable hot flashes, and there's even a risk of liver damage. So it's unwise to take without medical advice.

Soy to the Whirl

For a delicious, cholesterol-lowering shake, blend one cup of vanilla soy milk with two tablespoons of ground flaxseed. Add some fresh or frozen berries, and mix it all in the blender. The soy protein and flaxseed help lower LDLs and raise HDLs, while the berries add cholesterol-lowering fiber.

LDLs, decreasing your overall risk of heart disease and stroke. Plus, regular exercise helps control diabetes and high blood pressure, which are independent risk factors for heart disease.

A Capsule Summary

 ✎ If you aren't taking a prescription cholesterol-lowering drug, ask your doctor about **gugulipid supplements.** They seem to work by enabling the liver to take in more LDL, so that less of it circulates in the bloodstream. The usual dose is 75 milligrams of guggulsterones, the active ingredients in gugulipid (25 milligrams three times a day). Gugulipid is often combined with other cholesterol-lowering compounds such as **garlic, niacin**, and **red yeast rice extract.**

 ✎ Another alternative to prescription drugs is **red yeast rice extract.** It works by blocking an enzyme necessary to the formation of cholesterol and by speeding the removal of LDL from the blood. Follow the manufacturer's directions.

 ✎ Consider taking **artichoke extract.** Artichokes contain cynarin, a compound that increases the liver's production of bile—and bile plays a key role in the excretion of cholesterol from the body. Artichoke extract is available at health-food stores. Follow label instructions.

 ✎ Get your daily dose of **garlic**—either whole garlic or garlic pills. Garlic contains a compound called allicin, which is thought to be responsible for the herb's cholesterol-lowering effect. If you decide on garlic pills, look for enteric-coated tablets or capsules that provide a daily dose of at least 10 milligrams of alliin or a total allicin potential of 4,000 micrograms. (Alliin, one compound in garlic, converts into allicin inside the body.)

 ✎ Four times a day, take **ginger** capsules. The typical dose is 100 to 200 milligrams. Studies suggest that the compounds in ginger help to reduce the absorption and increase the excretion of LDL.

Hives

Asimple antihistamine can help reduce the allergic reaction causing your hives. Choose one of the newer drugs, such as Claritin or Alavert, that don't cause drowsiness. While you let the medicine do its work, try the handy home treatments below for added relief. You'll also want to get to the bottom of what's causing your hives so you can avoid itching in the future.

What's wrong

As small as jujubes or as large as saucers, hives are an allergic reaction that takes the form of itchy red bumps or welts on the skin. They are the result of cells releasing histamine, a chemical that makes blood vessels leak fluid into the deepest layers of skin. It's not clear why some people get hives, while others don't, and the "triggers" associated with hives are so numerous, they fit the category of "everything in the world." Just for starters, hives can be caused by sunlight, heat, cold, pressure, stress, viral infections, or medications. Name anything that can cause an allergy, and it can also cause hives—including pollen, dust, dander, dust mites, shellfish, and other foods.

Drown Them with Attention

 Unless you have hives that are triggered by cold (which is rare), take a **cool bath** or apply a **cold compress.** Cold shrinks the blood vessels and blocks further release of histamine. To further relieve itching, add **colloidal oatmeal** (like Aveeno) to the bathwater and soak for 10 to 15 minutes. (Be careful getting out of the tub, however—that fine-ground oatmeal turns slippery.)

A Dab Will Do

 Dab the welts with **calamine lotion** or **witch hazel.** These astringents help shrink blood vessels, so they don't leak so much histamine.

 Alternatives to calamine lotion are **milk of magnesia** or **Pepto-Bismol.** Because they are alkaline, they help to relieve the itching.

 In a small cup, add a few drops of water to **baking soda** and stir until you get a paste. Spread the paste on the hives to help stop irritation and relieve the itching.

 Do you have some **cream of tartar** in your kitchen cabinet? It might be just what you need to relieve the hives. Make a paste as above and apply.

 If you just have a few small hives and want to temporarily stop the itching, apply an over-the-counter **hydrocortisone cream.** Follow the directions on the package.

 Mix 1 teaspoon of any kind of **vinegar** with 1 tablespoon of lukewarm water and apply the mixture to your hives with a cotton ball or tissue to soothe the itching.

An old Chinese folk remedy for hives calls for boiling 2 ounces **brown sugar** and 1 ounce **fresh ginger** in 6 ounces **vinegar** for several minutes. Mix a little of the resulting liquid with warm water and apply several times per day.

Try a Common Weed

Herbalists recommend **nettle** as an alternative to antihistamines. Take up to six 400-milligram capsules a day. Or pick a few handfuls of the weed, steam, and eat. Wear gloves, long pants, and long sleeves to guard against nettle's stinging leaves.

Fish and the C

Take 1,000 milligrams of **fish oil** in capsule form three times a day. These capsules contain essential fatty acids that have anti-inflammatory properties. Cold-water fish like salmon, bluefish, and albacore tuna are good food sources.

Take 1,000 milligrams of **vitamin C** three times a day. At this dose, the "sunshine vitamin" has an effect that mimics the action of antihistamines. Don't take more than 1,000 milligrams a day or you might experience diarrhea.

Take Steps to Stop Stress

Stress can cause hives or make them worse. If your tension needs taming, master a nerve-calming technique such as **meditation, yoga**, or **progressive relaxation.**

Brew up a cup of **chamomile, valerian**, or **catnip tea.** All of these herbs have a sedative effect that may soothe your stress—and therefore your hives. To make the tea, stir one teaspoon of the dried herb into one cup of boiling water, steep 10 minutes, strain out the plant parts, and drink the tea.

Should I call **the doctor?**

While hives can be uncomfortable, they're usually harmless and disappear within minutes or hours. Sometimes they hang around for a few days. Seek emergency medical treatment if you develop hives around your eyes or in your mouth or experience difficulty breathing, wheezing, light-headedness, or dizziness. You may have a life-threatening condition called anaphylaxis, and the internal tissue swelling can block breathing passages. If you're prone to hives, ask your doctor if you should carry a rapid-injection form of epinephrine in case you develop anaphylaxis. And if you have chronic hives that just don't respond to milder treatments, your doctor may prescribe oral steroids.

Skin Graffiti

You probably don't think of your skin as a handy notepad, but if you have a hive condition called dermatographia, it could be. People who have dermatographia find that whenever they scratch or stroke their skin, they raise hivelike welts or swellings. That's because histamine and other chemicals are released in such a way to cause very localized redness, itchiness, and swelling. Often, people who develop dermatographia have no evidence of allergies, and the condition usually disappears without treatment—although, in some cases, antihistamines can help.

Did you **know?**

In their relentless hunt for causes of hives, doctors have discovered some very peculiar triggers. Some people get hives immediately after skin is exposed to water. Weirder still, hives can be triggered by exposure to something that's vibrating—such as the grip of a vacuum cleaner or the rapid vibration of an electric foot massager.

The Power of Prevention

To avoid hives, you need to figure out what causes them. If you don't know, start **keeping a daily diary**. The most probable suspects are things that you eat, drink, or swallow—food, drink, supplements, and medications. But even if you don't see any obvious connections, continue keeping your diary, noting other factors like weather, stress levels, clothing, or the amount of time that you spend in the sun. With careful tracking, you may link a specific lifestyle factor with the eruption of those red, itchy welts.

Foods most likely to trigger hives include **shellfish, nuts, chocolate, fish, tomatoes, eggs, fresh berries**, and **milk**. Some people react to preservatives in certain foods and wine, such as sulfites. Once you've identified a food trigger, eliminate it from your diet and see whether you have fewer outbreaks.

Common **drug triggers** include antibiotics and non-steroidal anti-inflammatory drugs (NSAIDs) such as aspirin and ibuprofen. But doctors have heard about many other triggers, including sedatives, tranquilizers, diuretics, diet supplements, antacids, arthritis medications, vitamins, eyedrops, eardrops, laxatives, and douches.

Impotence

As every man knows, numerous mental and physical factors influence the hydraulics. Once you've seen the doctor and crossed out the possibility of more serious health problems, you might want to take an all-points approach to erasing erectile dysfunction. That is, take up regular exercise and, at the same time, consider some of the mental factors that might be getting in the way—including boredom or anxiety in the bedroom. There are also some renowned herbs and supplements that might prove the key to more dependable arousal.

Help Diagnose the Problem

Healthy men normally have several erections during a night's sleep. Doctors have devices to test this, but here's a simple way to test on your own. Before going to sleep, take a **single-ply facial tissue**, cut a strip, and wrap it relatively tightly around your penis. Tape the end. If in the morning the tissue is torn, chances are you had a nocturnal erection. That's good news—it means you probably don't have an underlying physical problem to solve, but rather, psychological matters to deal with.

Stoke Your Fire with Herbs

Take **ginkgo**. It can improve blood flow in vessels throughout your body, including your penis. In one study, the herb helped men have erections even after a prescription injection didn't work. The recommended dose is 60 to 240 milligrams daily.

Try **Asian ginseng**, sometimes called Korean or Chinese ginseng. It's long been used to bolster male virility, since it can improve blood flow to the penis, reduce fatigue, and improve energy. Take 500 milligrams daily.

Look for botanical formulas that contain **suma, or Brazilian ginseng** (*Pfaffia*); **maca, or Peruvian ginseng** (*Lepidium*); and **muira puama** (also called **potency wood**). One formulation, called Sumacazon, produced by the Amazon Herb

What's **wrong**

An erection is the end result of a complex chain of events. The brain sends signals to the genitals, blood vessels dilate, and the penis gets engorged. Meanwhile, the veins that normally drain away blood get blocked. When a man cannot get or keep an erection, the problem is called impotence, or erectile dysfunction (ED). Common causes include clogged arteries, diabetes, and nerve problems. Depression, anxiety, and alcoholism can also be factors—in fact, roughly 30 percent of ED cases are psychologically caused. Many medications can be blamed as well, especially those used for high blood pressure and depression.

Should I call the doctor?

If your inability to have an erection lasts for more than two months or recurs frequently, talk to your doctor. You might be a good candidate for Viagra (or similar medication), and your doctor can outline the benefits and possible side effects. Also, in reviewing the medications that you're taking, your doctor might pinpoint some that are contributing to erectile dysfunction. And a physical examination might indicate that the erection problem is a sign of a more serious circulatory condition.

Company, contains all three. These Amazon rainforest herbs have been shown to enhance virility in both animals and humans.

Supplement Your Sexual Efforts

⌁ Buy **zinc** supplements and take 15 to 30 milligrams daily. This mineral increases production of testosterone, the hormone that's necessary for maintaining interest in sex.

⌁ Take **vitamin C.** It helps blood vessels stay flexible, allowing them to widen when you need more blood flow. You can take up to 1,000 milligrams three times a day. Cut back if you develop diarrhea.

⌁ Take a supplement containing 1,000 milligrams of **evening primrose oil** three times a day. The oil contains essential fatty acids that promote good blood vessel health. Alternatively, you can get these essential fatty acids by taking a tablespoon of flaxseed oil every morning.

⌁ The amino acid **arginine** can increase blood flow to the penis by increasing the production of nitric oxide in the blood vessel walls, improving artery flexibility and helping blood vessels dilate. The preferred form is L-arginine. Take two 750-milligram capsules twice daily between meals.

Don't Weigh Up

⌁ Get 30 minutes of **aerobic activity**—such as walking, jogging, swimming, or playing tennis—several days a week. Exercise helps keep excess weight off and keeps your heart and blood vessels healthier, including the ones that keep your penis operating properly.

Get Out of the Saddle

⌁ **If you're a bike rider, go easy.** Too much riding, or riding on the wrong saddle, can damage delicate nerves and blood vessels in the areas you sit on. Shop for a saddle that has a respectful groove running down the center. Be sure that your knees are slightly bent when your feet are at the bottom of each pedal cycle—this puts more of your weight *on* your legs instead of *between* them. Stand up at least every 10 minutes to let blood circulate to the genital area, and also level the pedals and stand up when you go over bumps to reduce jarring to your crotch.

Lose Tobacco to Keep Your Sex Life

☞ If you use tobacco in any form, **quit now.** Nicotine causes blood vessels to clamp down, impairing circulation. That means less blood can get to your penis.

Do Things Differently in the Bedroom

☞ If your erectile problems are due to stress and emotions rather than something physical, there are lots of ways to get yourself back in the game. For example, have bedroom intimacy **without having intercourse.** This takes off the pressure, relieving performance anxiety. Just hop in bed and cuddle, massage each other, or think of fun things to do that don't require an erection.

☞ Keep **variety in your activities.** Boredom with the same-old, same-old can hinder your ability to have an erection. Try new positions or do it elsewhere than in the bedroom. Check your bookstore or adult novelty store for books or games that offer suggestions.

☞ **Have sex in the morning.** You may have more spark since your testosterone level is higher at this time of day. Plus you shouldn't be as fatigued and frazzled as at the end of a long day.

Keep Up the Discussion

☞ If you keep the problem to yourself, you might be making it worse. Instead, **talk about it** with your partner. You can both brainstorm potential reasons why this may be happening— perhaps a bothersome disagreement or old aggravation is keeping you from performing properly. Not only will you find out your partner's point of view, you also benefit from having two people thinking of possible solutions.

☞ Let it go. Worrying about it too much will only make it worse. **Focus on other parts of your life** for a while, such as work, your hobbies, or your kids.

Should You Revise Your Rx's?

☞ Blood-pressure medications can contribute to erectile dysfunction, especially **beta-blockers** such as **metoprolol (Lopressor)** and **calcium channel blockers** such as **nifedipine (Procardia).** If you're taking these drugs, ask your

Skip it!

Alcohol helps relax you and stoke the fires of your desire, but it makes you less likely to be able to perform. Limit your consumption to two drinks a day or fewer.

Is It All in Your Mind—or Farther South?

Knowing if your erectile dysfunction is rooted in your mind or body will help you know how to solve it:

It's probably psychological if ... you still have erections sometimes—for example, when you wake up in the morning.

It's probably physical if... the problem came on gradually, and you have other problems in your genitals, such as difficulty urinating or numbness in your penis.

doctor if you can substitute something else that won't produce the same side effects.

🐛 Digitalis drugs for heart ailments, such as **digoxin (Lanoxin)**, can also present problems. But don't change the dosage until you have a chance to talk to your doctor.

🐛 Men taking certain antidepressant medications such as **Elavil, Prozac, Paxil,** and **Zoloft** frequently report erection problems. Since side effects are not predictable, your doctor may be able to "try you out" on a different antidepressant.

🐛 If you're taking the ulcer drug **Tagamet** and also experiencing erectile dysfunction, be sure to let your doctor know. This, too, is one of the common culprits.

Get Plenty of Rest and Relaxation

🐛 Try to get at least **six to eight hours** of sleep each night. Being fatigued definitely puts a damper on your ability to have an erection.

🐛 **Reduce your stress levels.** Anxiety and anger aren't conducive to the frame of mind needed for sex—plus, anxiety causes your body to make a form of adrenaline that interferes with the physical process behind an erection.

🐛 If you have trouble winding down, regularly engage in **meditation** or other forms of stress relief. For instance, you might spend a few minutes each day doing deep-breathing exercises—that is, just focusing on breathing in and out.

Indigestion

Great-Grandma and Great-Grandpa tamed their tummies with some of these comforting cures, and you may have luck with them too. No matter which teas or chewables you choose, though, you'll certainly want to cast a critical eye over the foods you eat—as well as how often and how much you munch. There's no free parking for the traffic in your GI tract. Once it's in, you pay the price.

Well-Rooted Traditions

⚬ **Ginger** is justifiably famous for settling stomach upset and improving digestion. You have three options: Take one or two 250-milligram capsules of ginger with meals, eat a few pieces of candied ginger as needed, or brew up a cup of ginger tea. To make the tea, stir 1 teaspoon grated gingerroot in 1 cup hot water, steep for 10 minutes, and strain.

⚬ **Chamomile**, an age-old treatment for indigestion. It calms the stomach and soothes spasms in the intestinal tract. Take a half-teaspoon chamomile tincture up to three times daily, or drink a few cups of chamomile tea throughout the day. Make it by stirring half to 1 teaspoon of dried herb into 1½ cups boiling water. Let it steep for 10 minutes, then strain and drink.

Pamper Yourself with Peppermint

⚬ **Peppermint oil** soothes intestinal muscle spasms and also helps relieve nausea. Take one or two capsules containing 0.2 milliliter of oil per capsule three times a day, between meals. Note that if you have heartburn, peppermint is *not* the cure for you.

⚬ If you'd prefer a steaming cup of **peppermint tea**, make it by steeping 1½ teaspoons of the dried herb in 1 cup hot water.

Chewable Resources

⚬ Chew and swallow a spoonful of **fennel** or **caraway seeds** when you're having indigestion (or you've eaten a big

What's **wrong**

The term "indigestion" covers a lot of ground, but mostly it means food isn't headed through your digestive tract smoothly and comfortably. Instead, you're experiencing nausea or possibly acid reflux as stomach acid backs up into your esophagus. Or maybe the problem is abdominal pain or bloating. There are many possible causes of indigestion, including eating too much or too quickly, eating foods that don't agree with you, and having too much or too little acid in your stomach.

Should I call **the doctor?**

If indigestion lasts for more than two weeks despite self-care approaches, talk to your doctor. Seek immediate medical attention if you have nausea accompanied by sweating or an ache in the chest; you may be having a heart attack. Other danger signs include abdominal pain that's accompanied by black or bloody stools or vomiting. (Black stools sometimes come from iron supplements or Pepto-Bismol, or from eating certain foods, but they may also be a sign of gastrointestinal bleeding.) Finally, call your doctor if you have any trouble eating, or if food won't go down.

or especially spicy meal that might cause indigestion). These seeds contain oils that soothe spasms in the gut, relieve nausea, and help control flatulence. That's why some Indian restaurants set out dishes of fennel seeds for customers.

⤷ Make a cup of **fennel tea.** Steep 2 to 3 teaspoons of crushed seeds in hot water for 10 minutes. Strain, then drink. You can also make the tea with anise seeds if you have them on hand.

⤷ Take **deglycyrrhizinated licorice, or DGL**, sold in health-food stores. This product soothes stomach upset and indigestion by coating the lining of the stomach. Chew the tablets as needed, following label directions.

Sour Solution

⤷ Try drinking 1 teaspoon of **apple cider vinegar** mixed with a half-cup of water, especially if you've overindulged in a large meal. It will help you digest the food if you don't have enough acid in your stomach. Add a little honey to sweeten the taste.

The Soda Solution

⤷ Stir a teaspoon of **baking soda** into a glass of water and drink it. If your stomach is too acidic, this solution neutralizes stomach acid and also helps relieve painful gas. Because in very rare cases baking soda can explode in the stomach and cause tears, some experts recommend adding a few drops of **lemon juice** to dispel some of the gas before it hits your stomach. (*Off-limits* … if you're on a low-sodium diet, since baking soda is high in sodium.)

Sip This

⤷ Some people claim that drinking a plain old cup of **hot water** eases indigestion.

⤷ Warm **ginger ale** or **lemon-lime soda**, or **flat Coca-Cola**, are also said to soothe an upset stomach.

Beware of Juice and Dairy

⤷ Though it's touted as a health drink, fruit juice can actually cause abdominal pain and gas. It contains fructose, a sugar that passes undigested into the colon. When bacteria in the colon finally break down the sugar, you're likely to get gas and bloating. If you drink juice, have **no more than 6 ounces** at a time, and drink it **with a meal** so you can digest it better.

If dairy foods make you feel gassy and bloated, the problem could be lactose intolerance—an inability to digest lactose, a sugar found in milk. To find out for sure, take this test: Drink 2 glasses of milk and see whether you get the symptoms that have been bothering you. If so, eliminate dairy foods from your diet or look for **lactose-free products** (or take a supplement containing **lactase**, the enzyme that digests lactose).

Eat Slowly, End Early

Eat slowly and deliberately. Wolfing down your food puts big chunks of material into your digestive system, and you also swallow air, which can contribute to bloating and flatulence. Plus, when you eat too fast, food doesn't get fully coated with saliva. That interferes with the digestive process.

Eat your last big meal of the day at least **three hours before bedtime.** You digest best when you're up and moving about, not while you're sleeping.

Tried...

Rubbing your belly can help relieve indigestion.

...and true
When you massage your lower abdomen, you push trapped gas and backed-up waste toward its natural exit. This can help put an end to bloating and constipation.

Inflammatory Bowel Disease

Doctors tend to treat IBD with powerful steroids and other prescription medications, and these drugs can be very helpful, especially during flare-ups. But there are steps you can take on your own to reduce the severity of your symptoms, such as favoring foods that are kind to your bowels and taking measures to manage stress.

What's **wrong**

The term "inflammatory bowel disease," or IBD, encompasses several conditions. The two most common ones are ulcerative colitis and Crohn's disease. Ulcerative colitis causes sores on the lining of the colon and rectum. Crohn's disease is more extensive—sometimes affecting the intestines, stomach, esophagus, and mouth—and tissues can become much more deeply inflamed. Symptoms are similar for both colitis and Crohn's: diarrhea, abdominal pain, and blood or mucus in the stool. These problems can flare up, then go away, with remissions sometimes lasting years.

Boost Beneficial Bacteria

⁓ Boost the population of beneficial bacteria in your gut. You can do this by taking an OTC bacteria supplement known as a **probiotic.** In healthy people, the colon is home to "good" bacteria (such as *Lactobacillus acidophilus* and *Bifidobacteria bifidum*) that prevent overgrowth of harmful bacteria. But when these bacteria are killed off—often, by antibiotics—the resulting overgrowth of "bad" bacteria and yeast can cause inflammation. Probiotics help maintain an optimal balance. If you don't want to take a supplement, try eating yogurt with active cultures.

Fuel Your Body with Care

⁓ Favor bland food—**cooked carrots, white rice, applesauce**, etc. If you're already suffering from diarrhea and abdominal pain, eating lots of spicy foods will only make matters worse.

⁓ **Cut back on dietary fat.** Fried foods, fatty meats, and other sources of fat can trigger contractions in your intestine, which can exacerbate diarrhea.

⁓ **Eat less dietary fiber** during flare-ups. Ordinarily, high-fiber foods like bran, whole grains, and broccoli are good for the system. But during flare-ups they increase your risk for painful gas. Once you feel better, resume a normal fiber intake.

⁓ Many people with Crohn's disease are unable to digest lactose, a form of sugar found in dairy foods. If you feel gassy and bloated, try **avoiding milk** and all other dairy foods for a few days. If your symptoms go away, you may have lactose intolerance. Switch to lactose-free dairy products, take pills containing lactase (the enzyme needed to digest milk), or avoid milk products altogether.

Track What You Eat

⮞ Keep a **food journal.** Record what foods you eat, what reactions you have, and the severity of your discomfort. At the end of a month, review your journal to get a sense of how well you tolerate dietary fiber and potentially troublesome foods like dairy products. You'll also find out whether you need to avoid any particular foods entirely.

Stress Less to Digest Best

⮞ Stress can trigger IBD symptoms. So every day, practice **yoga, meditation, deep breathing, visualization,** or another stress-reduction technique. For example, you might sit in a quiet spot for 20 minutes or so and visualize a healing blue light slowly pouring down the length of your digestive tract, soothing the inflammation. Imagine that as this blue light travels through you, it leaves healthy tissue behind.

Do Some Interior Work

⮞ Take a daily **multivitamin/mineral.** This helps restore the nutrients that can be depleted by persistent diarrhea.

⮞ A daily dose of a naturally occurring vitamin-like compound called **PABA (para-aminobenzoic acid)** may help ease inflammation within your intestines. During flare-ups, take 1,000 milligrams of PABA three times a day. Once your condition goes into remission, cut back to 1,000 milligrams twice a day. PABA is sold over the counter at drugstores.

⮞ Certain antioxidant nutrients help ease symptoms of IBD, although exactly why is unclear. Good choices include **grape-seed extract** (100 milligrams once or twice daily), the amino acid **NAC** (500 milligrams twice daily), and **vitamin C** (1,000 milligrams twice a day). All three are sold over the counter in drugstores.

⮞ Give the amino acid **L-glutamine** a try. An old folk remedy for intestinal inflammation calls for drinking lots of cabbage juice, which is rich in L-glutamine. But if that doesn't

Should I call the doctor?

If you have IBD, you should be under the care of a gastroenterologist. Alert the doctor if you experience a flare-up of symptoms, especially if you have diarrhea that contains blood or mucus. That could be an indication of cancer or another potentially life-threatening condition.

sound particularly appetizing, you can simply take L-glutamine pills (500 milligrams a day). L-glutamine helps heal ulcers in the gut.

Because it combats inflammation, a type of **licorice** called **DGL** may help ease symptoms of inflammatory bowel disease. Chew two wafers (380 milligrams) three times a day between meals when you have a flare-up. Don't try to substitute licorice candy; most licorice candy contains no "real" licorice. And unlike DGL, "real" licorice can raise your blood pressure.

Oil Your Inflammation Away

Omega-3 fatty acids are essential for good digestion. Good sources include **flaxseed oil** (one tablespoon a day taken straight or mixed into salad dressing or cereal) and **fish oil** (1,500 milligrams to 3,000 milligrams of fish-oil capsules daily). One Italian study found that fish oil reduced the frequency of intestinal attacks in people with Crohn's disease.

Teatime Again

Peppermint and **chamomile** contain antispasmodic compounds that help curb cramps and ease pain caused by abdominal gas. To make a tea, drop a teaspoon of either dried herb into a cup of boiling water, and let it steep for 10 minutes. Strain and drink. If you're susceptible to heartburn, choose chamomile over peppermint.

Marshmallow tea soothes by coating the mucous membranes in the digestive tract. Use 1 to 2 teaspoons of dried herb per cup of hot water. Steep for 10 to 15 minutes, then strain.

Insect and Spider Bites

If you live near a polar ice cap, you'll never have to worry about mosquitoes, bees, wasps, or spiders. For the rest of us, confrontations with these pesky predators are as inevitable as the summer solstice. For some bugs, insect repellent is an effective deterrent. Others, however, seem eternally bold, and their bites are as bad as their buzz. Here's how to recover from sneak attacks and protect your skin from further affronts.

WASP AND BEE STINGS

Get Out the Credit Card

If you've been stung by anything larger than a mosquito (a honeybee, for instance), **scrape away the stinger** as soon as possible using the edge of a credit card, a knife blade, or your fingernail. As long as it remains in your skin, this little sac of poison keeps pumping its contents into your body. Don't use tweezers or pinch the stinger with your fingertips, since you'll squeeze more venom into your skin.

Pamper the Sting Site

As soon as you have the stinger out, soak the area in **apple cider vinegar** for a few minutes. Dip a cotton ball in vinegar and tape it to the sting site. It will help relieve redness and swelling.

Treat the area with **meat tenderizer** right after you're stung. It contains enzymes that break down the venom, reducing swelling and inflammation. Take a few spoonfuls of meat tenderizer powder, add enough water to form a paste, smear the paste on, and leave it on for an hour.

Apply an **aspirin paste** to stop the itching. Using the back of a spoon, crush one or two aspirins on a small plate or cutting board. Add just enough water to make a paste, then dab the paste on the sting site. Ingredients in aspirin help to neutralize the venom.

Apply an **ice pack** to numb the area and help slow the

What's **wrong**

Some bugs bite you because they're hungry and they see you as food. Mosquitoes, ticks, fleas, and chiggers are on this team. Others sting you because they regard you as a threat. This club includes spiders, wasps, fire ants, yellow jackets, and bees. Mosquitoes inject you with a little saliva that leaves a maddeningly itchy bump, while bees and wasps penetrate skin with a poison that makes you yelp and run. Worst, of course, are venomous spiders—but fortunately, they're the rarest of foes.

If you know you've been bitten by a spider, try to memorize its appearance. Some spiders can cause serious symptoms affecting your whole body, while others just create a localized reaction. Whether or not you have a severe reaction, get medical attention right away.

Should I call **the doctor?**

If you've been bitten by a spider, call the doctor immediately. If you've been stung by a bee or wasp and then have trouble breathing, feel faint, or have swelling in your mouth or throat, a rapid pulse, or hives, get to an emergency room. You could be having a potentially fatal allergic reaction called anaphylaxis. And see a doctor if you develop a bull's-eye rash, muscle aches, fever, and headache within three weeks after getting a tick bite; these could be signs of Lyme disease, which can lead to mental confusion and arthritis if not treated.

swelling. If you have a towel or washcloth between the ice pack and your skin, you can leave the ice pack in place for up to 20 minutes.

Papaya contains enzymes that neutralize insect venom. If you happen to have this fruit in your lunch basket, simply lay a slice on the sting for an hour.

Baking soda can bring relief. One method of application is to mix baking soda with a skin lotion, then apply it to the sensitive area. The baking soda helps relieve inflammation, and the skin lotion keeps it in place. Alternatively, you can mix one teaspoon of baking soda in a glass of water, let it dissolve, then apply the mixture with a cotton pad or washcloth. Leave the compress in place for 20 minutes.

Cut an **onion**, then rub it over the sting site. Doctors aren't quite sure how this works, but the onion contains enzymes that seem to break down inflammatory compounds. Other people swear by smearing a crushed clove of **garlic** over the skin.

Sugar works too. Just dip your forefinger in water, dab it in sugar, then touch the sting site.

To help reduce swelling, try **bromelain**, a protein-digesting enzyme derived from pineapple. On an empty stomach take 500 milligrams containing at least 2,000 GDU or 3,000 MCU. You can take several doses in a single day. Stop taking it when the swelling goes down.

Tea-tree oil will also help reduce the swelling. Apply one drop several times a day.

To stop the itching, dab on a drop or two of **lavender oil**. Wait about 15 minutes to allow the oil to take effect. If the area starts to itch again, apply more—but just one or two drops at a time.

Outsmart Ticks' Tricks

If you've been in tick territory, be sure to follow this advice.

🔹 After you've been in the woods or weeds, strip off your clothes and check yourself from head to toe. (Have your spouse or partner check parts of your body you can't see.)

🔹 If you find a tick that hasn't attached to your skin, grasp it with a napkin or piece of toilet paper, and flush it down the toilet.

🔹 If a tick has already latched onto your skin, use tweezers to grab it by the head, as close to your skin as possible. Slowly pull upward until it lets go. If you yank it off, the head can break off in your skin and remain there until infection sets in.

🔹 Preserve any tick that has been embedded in your skin in a zipped-up plastic sandwich bag. If you develop a rash, your doctor can analyze the tick to see whether it carries Lyme disease. A rash can show up from three days to a month later, so keep that bagged tick for a while before flushing it away.

INSECT BITES

Instead of Scratching...

🔹 Rub an **ice cube** on the bug bite right away. This helps decrease the inflammation that causes itching.

🔹 **Sea Breeze astringent** for oily skin will stop the itching from mosquito bites. In addition to alcohol, its contents include camphor, eucalyptus, clove oil, eugenol, and peppermint oil. Dab a small amount on a cotton pad or tissue, and apply it to the site.

🔹 **Underarm deodorants** have ingredients that reduce skin irritation. If you get a bug bite, try any deodorant and see if it works.

🔹 Apply a drop or two of **peppermint oil**. It has a cooling effect, and also increases circulation to the bite, speeding the healing process. Alternatively, if you have toothpaste that contains peppermint oil, apply a dab.

🔹 Look for an anti-itch spray or gel that contains **menthol**, a classic skin-soother. Keep the product in the refrigerator until you're ready to use it. The coolness will provide extra itch relief.

🔹 Buy anti-itch cream that contains a topical anesthetic to numb the area. Some also contain **hydrocortisone** to stop the swelling and **antihistamine** to counter the allergic reaction.

🔹 Use a **bug-bite relief patch**, which looks like a small bandage and goes directly on the skin. Each patch contains concentrated numbing medicine.

Skip it!

Tick bite? Smearing the tick with petroleum jelly or oil won't cause it to come loose, as some would have you believe. Removing the head with tweezers is the effective way to get the job done.

The Power of Prevention

Use a bug spray that contains **DEET**, the most effective insect repellent for use on the skin. Adults can safely use any DEET product (following directions on the label). Children should not be exposed to a cream that exceeds 6% DEET.

Before heading into the deep woods, treat your clothing with one of the many insect repellents that contain **permethrin**. Permethrin is a synthetic version of a bug-repelling compound found in chrysanthemum plants. Apply it liberally to outdoor-wear clothing, and it should remain effective even after a washing. Permethrin only goes on clothing, but not for safety reasons: The compound loses its effectiveness when it's applied to skin.

You can also use products made with **p-Menthane 3, 8-diol**, a chemical derived from the eucalyptus plant. **Off! Botanicals** is one product that contains this ingredient.

Citronella, an oil that comes from a type of grass, is found in bug-repelling candles, as well as bug sprays. Follow label directions.

Several days before you take a camping or hiking trip into bug-filled territory, start eating **garlic**. Have a clove or two every day. As you sweat out the garlic odor, it repels many insects.

To **keep bees away**, avoid wearing perfumes or scented products, keep food and soda covered, and don't wear bright clothing, especially floral patterns.

Insomnia

Insomnia can become a real nightmare as the clock ticks on into the night and you're awake to notice. What to do? Try counting sheep. Seriously. If that doesn't work, you could follow Mark Twain's advice: "Lie near the edge of the bed and you'll drop off." Better yet, try the other approaches listed below. A relaxing cup of tea, a whiff of lavender oil, smarter scheduling of sleep, and other tactics can summon the sandman and help you awaken less tired and cranky come morning.

Before-Bed Bites

    Have a slice of **turkey** or **chicken**, or a **banana** before heading to bed. These foods contain tryptophan, an amino acid that's used to make serotonin. And serotonin is a brain chemical that helps you sleep. Keep the portion small, though, or your full belly may keep you awake.

    Carbohydrates help trytophan enter the brain. Try a glass of **warm milk** (milk contains tryptophan) and a **cookie**, or warm milk with a spoonful of **honey**. A sprinkling of **cinnamon** couldn't hurt, and might add mild sedative properties of its own.

    Avoid big meals late in the evening. You need three to four hours to digest a big meal, so if you eat a lot within four hours of your bedtime, don't be surprised if intestinal grumblings and groanings keep you awake.

    Spicy or sugary food, even at suppertime, is usually a bad idea. **Spices can irritate your stomach**, and when it tosses and turns, so will you. Having a lot of sugary food—especially chocolate, which contains caffeine—can make you feel jumpy.

Call on Herbs for Help

    Valerian helps people fall asleep faster without the "hangover" affect of some sleeping pills. It binds to the same receptors in the brain that tranquilizers such as Valium bind to. The herb itself stinks (think sweaty old socks), so we don't

What's wrong

Insomnia can take three forms: (1) You toss and turn instead of falling asleep; (2) You fall asleep okay, but then wake up repeatedly during the night; or (3) You wake up too early and can't fall asleep again. Whatever the form of sleep thievery, you've been set up for grogginess and irritability the next day. The most common causes of insomnia are emotional stress and depression. Other reasons for poor sleep include pain or illness, medications (such as decongestants), eating a heavy meal late at night, drinking caffeine or alcohol too near bedtime, or simply trying to sleep in an unfamiliar bed.

Should I call
the doctor?

If you've tried the following self-care strategies and still can't get a good night's sleep, talk to your doctor. And waste no time getting to your doctor if sleep deprivation is harming your work performance or endangering your life—as in, causing you to fall asleep at the wheel. You may need to be evaluated overnight at a sleep clinic.

recommend trying to make a tea. Instead, take one-half to one teaspoon of valerian tincture or two capsules of valerian root an hour before bed.

Take 4,000 to 8,000 milligrams of dried **passionflower** capsules. Passionflower is widely used as a mild herbal sedative.

Or you can combine forces, taking a supplement that includes both **passionflower** and **valerian**. "Natural" sleep remedies often include other herbal ingredients as well, such as **hops** and **skullcap**. Whatever the formulation, follow the package directions.

Smell Your Way to Sleep

Lavender has a reputation as a mild tranquilizer. Simply dab a bit of the oil onto your temples and forehead before you hit the pillow. The aroma should help send you off to sleep. You can also add lavender oil to a diffuser or vaporizer to scent your bedroom. Or place a lavender sachet near your pillow.

Put a drop of **jasmine** essential oil on each wrist just before you go to bed. In studies conducted at Wheeling Jesuit University in West Virginia, researchers discovered that people who spent the night in jasmine-scented rooms slept more peacefully than people who stayed in unscented—or even lavender-scented—rooms.

Try a soothing aromatic **bath** before bedtime. Add 5 drops **lavender oil** and 3 drops **ylang-ylang oil** to warm bathwater and enjoy a nice soak.

Be a Slave to Schedule

Wake up at the same time each day, no matter how little sleep you got the night before. On weekends, follow the same schedule, so your body adheres to the same pattern all week long. You'll fall asleep faster.

Every morning, **go for a walk**. It doesn't have to be a long walk, but it should definitely be outdoors. The presence of natural light (even if the day is overcast) tells your groggy body it's time to wake up for the day. With your body clock set by the great outdoors, you'll sleep better at night.

Try not to nap during the day, no matter how tired you feel. People who don't have insomnia often benefit from a short afternoon nap. However, if you're napping in daytime only to turn into a wide-eyed zombie at night, there's a good chance that that afternoon snooze is disrupting your body clock. If you absolutely must nap, catch a half-hour of zzz's at the most.

Pillow Tricks

🍂 Once you get into bed, imagine your feet becoming heavy and numb. Feel them sinking into the mattress. Then do the same with your calves, and slowly work your way up your body, letting it all grow heavy and relaxed. The idea is to **let yourself go**, in gradual phases, all the way from head to toe.

🍂 If you're still awake after this progressive relaxation exercise, **count sheep**. Sound like an old saw? The whole point is to occupy your mind with boring repetition, and, not to cast aspersions on sheep, there's nothing more boring or repetitive than counting a herd of them. Any repetitive counting activity will lull you.

🍂 If you prefer lullabies, listen to **calming, relaxing tapes** as you drift off.

🍂 If you just can't sleep, **don't lie in bed worrying about it**. That will only make sleep harder to attain. Get up, leave the bedroom, and grab a book or watch TV. Recommended reading, at this time of night, is some mind-numbing tome about the history of Swiss watch-making or macroeconomic theory. And if you decide to watch TV, look for a channel showing coverage of a recent zoning-board hearing or something equally soporific. The goal is to bore yourself into oblivion—so sleep becomes a sweet release.

Prep Your Bedroom

🍂 If you find yourself tossing and turning as you try to get comfortable, consider purchasing a special **neck-supporting pillow**. They are specially designed for people who have neck pain or tension that prevents sleep.

🍂 **Turn your alarm clock** so that you **can't see it** from bed. If you're glancing at the clock when you wake up—and it's almost impossible not to—you'll soon start wondering how you can function tomorrow on so little sleep tonight. For truly

Tried...

A hops pillow can help relieve insomnia.

...and true

Hops—flowers of a plant used in beer-making—release a mild sedative into the air. To make your own pillow, sew two 8-inch squares of fabric together along three sides to form a pocket. Stuff it full of dried hops and sew the fourth side shut. Put the pillow near your head so you can smell it at night. You may need to periodically dampen it with grain alcohol to reactivate the herb.

Skip it!

Avoid sleep inducers containing kava. Though derivatives of this plant root reduce anxiety and relax your muscles, kava supplements have been linked to liver toxicity in recent years. They have been pulled off the market in many countries.

accomplished insomniacs, just one glance at a glowing digital dial is enough to set a whole anxiety-train in motion.

 Turn your thermostat down a few degrees before heading to bed. Most people sleep better when their surroundings are cool.

 If you share your bed, consider buying a **queen- or king-size mattress** so you don't keep one another up. Some new models are designed so that when your partner moves—or if a bowling ball drops on his or her side of the bed—you feel nothing. Or consider sleeping in separate beds. (If you value the relationship, of course, be sure to emphasize that your wish for separate beds is based on pragmatism rather than preference.)

Check the Label

 Be cautious about taking an over-the-counter painkiller before bed. Some of them, like Excedrin, contain **caffeine**. Read the label first.

 Check labels of decongestants and cold remedies too. In addition to caffeine, they may contain ingredients, such as pseudoephedrine, that rev up your nervous system and leave you unable to fall asleep. Look for a **nighttime formula**.

Don'ts and More Don'ts for Better Dozing

 Avoid exercising within four hours of bedtime—it's too stimulating. Instead, exercise in the morning or after work. An exception is **yoga**. A number of yoga postures are designed to calm your body and prepare you for sleep.

 Avoid caffeinated beverages, particularly within four hours of bedtime. Though people have varying ranges of sensitivity to caffeine, the stimulating effects can be long-lasting.

 Also **avoid alcohol** in the evenings. While a glass of sherry might help you fall asleep a bit faster than usual, the effects soon wear off, and you're more likely to wake up during the night.

 If you **smoke** within four hours of your bedtime, look no further for the **cause of your insomnia**. Nicotine stimulates the central nervous system, interfering with your ability to fall asleep and stay that way.

Irritable Bowel Syndrome

Since there's no sure cure for IBS (also called "spastic colon"), people develop their own ways of living with the enemy. The key: Don't become discouraged. Dietary changes and stress-relief tactics should provide a significant dose of relief. For more insurance, combine them with one of the alternative therapies noted below. Once you have a system for controlling your symptoms, IBS will surely put less of a cramp in your style.

Cut the Stress Connection

‹ Since stress is one of the factors known to trigger an IBS flare-up, learn to short-circuit it with **meditation**, **yoga**, or a **simple breathing exercise** like this one. Sit comfortably, or lie down. Turn your attention to the air going in and out of your body. When upsetting or anxiety-producing thoughts intrude, focus completely on your breathing. Practice this daily. Then, whenever you feel yourself becoming tense and anxious, use it to calm yourself.

‹ **Keep a diary** of your IBS symptoms, noting what types of problems you have and how severe they are. In this journal, also jot down any stressful events you face in your day. Occasionally look back at your diary. If you see more IBS symptoms just before airplane flights or meetings with your boss, for instance, there may be a connection. Once you've detected situations that seem to trigger IBS symptoms, look for ways—like using the breathing technique above—to cope with them better.

Go Easy on Your Intestines

‹ **Minimize fried foods, meats, oils, margarine, dairy foods,** and **other fatty foods.** They cause your colon to contract violently, which can lead to diarrhea and abdominal pain.

‹ **Stay away from spicy foods.** The capsaicin in hot peppers, for example, makes your large intestine go into spasms, which can cause diarrhea.

What's wrong

Normally, food travels through your digestive system propelled by wavelike contractions of the intestinal muscles. But if you have irritable bowel syndrome, or IBS, the contractions are irregular—fast and spastic, causing diarrhea, or slow and weak, causing constipation. Other symptoms include abdominal pain and gas. Causes are unknown, but doctors have discovered that elevated stress, along with certain foods, aggravate IBS. Women are twice as likely as men to get the syndrome.

Should I call **the doctor?**

Call your doctor if you notice blood in your stool, you start losing weight when you're not trying to, or your IBS symptoms are so severe that you can't even leave your home. If you're over 50 and start to have IBS symptoms, you should get a doctor involved. And if you've had IBS for many years but note a change in a previous pattern, make the call. Among other things, the doctor should ask you about prescription or OTC medications to find out whether a change in bowel habits is related to drug side effects.

✒ **Cut down on caffeine.** It can worsen IBS by irritating your intestines.

✒ **Avoid** foods known to cause flatulence, including **cabbage, Brussels sprouts,** and **broccoli.**

✒ **Don't chew gum or candy that contains artificial sweeteners.** Among the common sweeteners in these products are **sorbitol** and **mannitol,** which can have a laxative effect. They're very difficult to digest. When bacteria in your colon eventually break down these "nonabsorbed sugars," you get gas and diarrhea.

✒ **Stop smoking.** Nicotine contributes to IBS flare-ups. Also, when you smoke, you swallow air, and people with IBS are very sensitive to having air in their gut.

Fit In More Fiber

✒ Soluble fiber soaks up liquid in your intestines, helping to prevent diarrhea. Good sources are **beans, oatmeal,** and some **fruits,** such as **apples, strawberries,** and **grapefruit.**

✒ If you can't seem to get enough soluble fiber in your diet, take a daily supplement of **psyllium,** the main ingredient in dietary fiber supplements like Metamucil. Unlike chemical laxatives, psyllium is safe to take long-term. Follow the label for dosage directions.

✒ If constipation is your main complaint, fill up on **insoluble fiber,** found in **whole wheat, bran,** other **whole grains, salad greens,** and other foods. Insoluble fiber bulks up stool, which speeds its passage through the intestines.

✒ If you haven't had much fiber in your diet, **increase the amount you eat gradually.** Adding too much fiber all at once can actually give you gas and bloating. Start with 8 grams of fiber daily—about what you'd find in two pears—and increase by 3 or 4 grams each day until you're up to 30 grams daily.

Cowed by Dairy?

Many people who think they have IBS actually have lactose intolerance, a problem in which the body can't properly digest the lactose sugar that's found in dairy foods. An easy way to self-diagnose this is to drink two eight-ounce glasses of milk. If you are lactose intolerant, you will get cramps, gas, and diarrhea. If you get these symptoms, you know it's time to drop all dairy foods from your diet. Instead of pouring milk on your cereal in the morning, use Lactaid, which is almost entirely lactose-free.

➤ Drink at least six to eight glasses of **water** each day to keep fiber moving smoothly through your system.

Graze, Don't Gorge

➤ Eat **smaller meals** more frequently rather than a couple of large meals each day. Taking in too much food at once can overstimulate your digestive system.

➤ If you usually bolt down your meals, **go more slowly** and pay more attention to chewing your food. Fast eaters often swallow too much air, which turns into bothersome intestinal gas.

Eat Yogurt

➤ Having diarrhea can drain away good bacteria that help prevent harmful bacteria from growing out of control. When you're having IBS-related diarrhea, eat plenty of **yogurt** containing active bacteria, such as acidophilus. Or take supplements of **acidophilus**. The usual daily dosage is one pill containing 1 billion to 2 billion live organisms. Take it on an empty stomach.

Steep Well

➤ Every day, drink a cup or two of **peppermint tea**, which relaxes your intestines, reduces spasms, and relieves gas pain. Make sure to buy the kind that contains real peppermint, rather than black tea with peppermint flavoring. (*Off-limits* . . . if you have heartburn.) Alternatively, you can take enteric-coated **peppermint-oil** capsules. The coating ensures that the oil reaches the intestine instead of breaking down in the stomach. Take one or two capsules three times a day, between meals.

➤ Drink **ginger tea**. Ginger soothes all manner of digestive problems, including IBS. For the freshest tea, grate a half-teaspoon of ginger into a cup, then pour in hot water, let it steep for 10 minutes, strain out the ginger, and drink the tea. Ginger tea bags are also available. Drink four to six cups a day.

Exorcise with Exercise

➤ Whenever possible, get at least 30 minutes of non-competitive **exercise** such as walking. Exercise helps relieve stress, releases natural painkilling endorphins, and keeps your body—including your digestive system—working smoothly.

Skip it!

Avoid using medications to affect your bowel habits—either laxatives for constipation or drugs to fight diarrhea—if you have IBS. These can make you swing wildly back and forth between constipation and diarrhea.

Kidney Stones

It's been said that the pain of passing a kidney stone is comparable to that of giving birth. Whether that's true or not, you'll probably want to stay home and take over-the-counter pain relievers to take the edge off this experience. You can also place a hot-water bottle over the painful area to provide some measure of relief. After that, it's a waiting game. The stones might pass in a few hours, but sometimes it takes days. Fortunately, you can take measures to speed up the process a little.

What's wrong

The pain in your back and side is so excruciating that you feel as if you might vomit. The cause: a nasty nugget formed from crystals that separate from the urine and build up on the inner surfaces of the kidney. Now that tiny stone wants to exit via the ureter, the spaghetti-thin tube that empties the bladder. Up to 80 percent of stones are made of calcium in combination with oxalate or phosphate. Less common are stones composed of uric acid or cystine. Heredity, chronic dehydration, repeated urinary tract infections, and a sedentary lifestyle are all thought to contribute to kidney stone formation.

Flush It Out

To flush the stone into the bladder, drink at least **three quarts of water** a day. If you're gulping enough water to do the job, your urine should run clear, with not a trace of yellow.

During an attack, drink as much **dandelion tea** as you can. A strong diuretic, dandelion stimulates blood circulation through the kidneys, increasing urine output and helping to flush out the stone. To make the tea, add 2 teaspoons dried herb to 1 cup boiling water. Steep for 15 minutes, then drink.

Consider drinking two or three cups daily of **corn silk, buchu,** or **couch grass tea.** Like dandelion, these herbals have diuretic properties to help flush out and prevent kidney stones.

Stepping Stone

When you have a kidney stone, the slightest move is likely to be painful. But if you can bear to **take a walk,** try to do it. Walking may jar the stone loose. Despite the discomfort, you might pass the stone more quickly if you just keep moving.

An Old Saw

As soon as you have symptoms of a kidney stone, take two 160-milligram capsules of **saw palmetto.** If the stone does not pass right away, continue taking the same daily dose until it does. The blue-black fruit of the saw palmetto, which has been called "plant catheter" and "old man's friend," has long been used as a home remedy for urinary and prostate problems.

Saw palmetto relaxes the ureter, which makes it easier to pass a stone.

The Power of Prevention

⁓ Many experts believe that the single most important thing you can do to prevent kidney stones is the same thing you do to make them pass more quickly—that is, drink enough fluids. Anyone who is prone to kidney stones should drink at least **8 to 10 cups of water a day**, every day. The more you drink, the more you dilute the substances that form stones.

⁓ Stick to a **low-sodium diet** to reduce the calcium in your urine, which may reduce your risk of forming new stones. A good start: Limit your consumption of fast foods, canned soups, and other processed foods. The target is less than 2,400 milligrams of sodium a day.

⁓ Drink two 8-ounce glasses of **cranberry juice** each day. Research suggests that it may help reduce the amount of calcium in the urine. In a study of people with calcium stones, cranberry juice reduced the amount of calcium in the urine by 50 percent.

⁓ If you don't like cranberry juice, drink **orange juice** or **lemonade**—6 ounces at each meal. The citric acid these juices contain will raise the citrate level in your urine, helping to keep new calcium stones from forming.

⁓ **Magnesium** has been shown to prevent all types of kidney stones. Eat more foods rich in this mineral, such as dark-green leafy vegetables, wheat germ, and seafood. You can also take 800 milligrams a day in supplement form.

⁓ Ramp up your intake of fruits and vegetables, which are rich in **potassium**. In studies, people who ate a lot of produce

Should I call **the doctor?**

Most stones pass without a doctor's help, but the first time you get one, it's inevitable that you'll call the doctor. With pain like this, you definitely want to report your symptoms. They include nausea and vomiting, bloody or cloudy urine, needing to urinate but not being able to, a burning sensation upon urination, or fever and chills (which may indicate infection). Even if you've had kidney stones before, call your doctor if the pain becomes excruciating. Severe cases may require hospitalization and narcotic painkillers.

Strain and Tell

As distasteful as it may sound, most experts recommend that during an acute attack, folks with kidney stones urinate through a piece of gauze, cheesecloth, or a fine-mesh strainer. Why? So you can catch a stone, should you pass one, and take it to your doctor. The doctor will have it analyzed to find out whether it's composed of calcium oxalate, calcium phosphate, uric acid, or other substances. Based on that analysis, you can make specific dietary changes to prevent a recurrence.

slashed their risk of kidney stones by half. If you suffer from stones regularly, ask your doctor whether potassium supplements might help you ward off future attacks.

⤙ **Cut back on coffee.** Caffeine increases calcium in the urine, which increases the risk of stone formation.

⤙ If you know your stones are made of calcium oxalate (a urine test can tell you), **cut back on foods rich in oxalates.** These foods include spinach, chocolate, wheat bran, nuts (especially peanuts), strawberries, and raspberries. Also avoid black tea, which is high in oxalates.

⤙ If you have had uric-acid stones in the past, you need to keep your urine as alkaline as possible to prevent a recurrence. **Avoid foods that raise acid levels,** including anchovies, sardines, organ meats, and brewer's yeast. Also, don't eat more than 3 ounces of meat or more than one serving of oatmeal, tuna, ham, lima beans, or spinach a day.

⤙ **Calcium** in the diet may help prevent calcium oxalate stones, probably because calcium combines with oxalate in the intestine and so prevents the body's absorption of pure oxalate. Foods rich in calcium include milk, cheese, yogurt, dark green leafy vegetables, nuts, and seeds. Taking calcium supplements during or just after meals may have a similar effect, but taking them between meals can increase the risk of stones.

Menopause Problems

You may feel as if your body is out of control and you never know what unpleasant surprise it may hold in store for you. Maybe you awaken in the middle of the night drenched in sweat, or you suffer from irritability, annoying mental "fuzziness," and memory lapses. First, remember that menopause doesn't last forever. Then try these approaches for relief in the meantime.

Say Yes to Soy

🔹 Eat 6 to 8 ounces of **tofu** every day. Tofu is high in phytoestrogens—compounds with mild estrogen-like qualities that have been found to ease menopausal symptoms. Certain kinds of phytoestrogens, called isoflavones, found in soy products can help ease hot flashes and vaginal dryness. The recommended amount is 60 milligrams a day of isoflavones, which is what you'll get by eating 6 to 8 ounces of tofu.

🔹 One 50-milligram supplement of **isoflavones**, taken daily, can meet most of your needs when you can't eat a lot of tofu. Look for brands that contain genistein and daidzein. One widely available brand, Promensil, has both of these components and is often recommended by doctors.

🔹 **Flaxseeds** are another source of phytoestrogens. Grind some in a spice grinder and add 1 to 2 tablespoons to cereal or yogurt.

Don't Sweat It

🔹 To help control hot flashes and night sweats, take ½ to 1 milliliter of **black cohosh** in tincture form two to four times a day. To make it more palatable, add the tincture to half a glass of juice or water. Research has shown that the herb helps control hot flashes by lowering blood levels of luteinizing hormone (LH), which dilates blood vessels and sends heat to the skin. You might get other benefits as well, since some women have found that black cohosh can relieve vaginal dryness, nervousness, and depression. For maximum

What's **wrong**

A woman is officially done with menopause when she hasn't menstruated for one year. But in the years preceding menopause, called perimenopause, her ovaries are producing less of the female sex hormones estrogen and progesterone, while ovulation (the monthly release of an egg) also becomes less frequent. This hormonal ebb can result in a variety of uncomfortable symptoms, including hot flashes and night sweats, vaginal dryness, mood swings, sleep problems, and unusually light or heavy periods.

Should I call the doctor?

Menopause isn't a disease, of course. It's a milestone. And some women don't even have symptoms. But many women do, and the discomfort can run the gamut from mildly annoying to extremely bothersome. If you're experiencing changes in your cycle—like irregular periods or unusual flow—see your doctor to make sure the changes are related to menopause and not a medical problem. If you have urinary discomfort, see a doctor to check for bladder infections, which occur more frequently among women who have vaginal dryness. Also, schedule an appointment if you miss a period or you develop vaginal bleeding between periods, or if you just don't feel like yourself because of your symptoms.

effectiveness, take black cohosh for 6 weeks, then take four weeks off before resuming it again. Then repeat the cycle—6 weeks on, 4 weeks off.

⌐ To tame night sweats, take 3 to 15 drops **sage tincture** three times a day in a half-cup water or tea. The genus name of this herb, *Salvia,* comes from the Latin *salvere* (to heal), and the extract of salvia leaves has been used to treat more than 60 different health complaints. The herb has astringent qualities that can help quell profuse sweating.

⌐ Some women find that taking **vitamin E** can help to relieve hot flashes and night sweats as well as mood swings and vaginal dryness. The recommended dose is 800 milligrams a day (400 milligrams twice a day). Consult your doctor before you start taking it regularly. This is especially important if you have diabetes, bruise easily, or have high blood pressure.

⌐ To help stay cool, wear lightweight clothing made of **natural fibers**. And carry a small, battery-powered **fan** with you to cool off the hot flashes.

⌐ Some women find that taking a **tepid bath** in the morning for 20 minutes prevents hot flashes all day long.

Exert Yourself

⌐ Increase the amount of **aerobic exercise** you get until you're getting at least 20 minutes a day. Besides helping you lose weight, exercise has other positive effects for women going through menopause. Studies show that daily vigorous physical activity decreases hot flashes and night sweats, helps improve mood and sleep, and improves the balance of hormone levels. Weight-bearing activities like walking, running, and resistance training also help keep your bones sturdy.

A Liver Saver

If you take synthetic hormones, you might have symptoms related to excess hormone levels—such as breast tenderness, bloating, or headaches. But some of these symptoms can be alleviated with milk thistle, an herb that helps the liver clear away some byproducts from the synthetic hormones. Milk thistle also helps repair and regenerate liver cells. The recommended dose is 420 milligrams a day in divided doses. Take that amount for 6 to 8 weeks, then taper down to 280 milligrams a day in divided doses.

Stay Chaste

✐ The berries of the **chaste tree** have been used by women for some 2,000 years. They help restore progesterone levels, which decrease significantly during menopause. Chaste tree may be particularly useful for combating very heavy bleeding, which some women experience during perimenopause. It may also help with other symptoms, including hot flashes and depression. Take 1 to 2 teaspoons of a standardized extract once a day.

Meal Plans

✐ If you've been getting hot flashes, **stay away from alcohol, coffee, spicy foods**, and **hot drinks**. Many of these foods are triggers.

✐ To help prevent accelerating bone loss—osteoporosis—make sure you get enough **protein**. It doesn't take much chicken, fish, or meat to supply your daily requirement for protein. As long as you have a serving that's about equal to the size of a deck of cards, you're getting enough. Also make sure you get 1,500 to 2,000 milligrams of **calcium** per day plus **vitamin** D. Low-fat dairy products are good sources. A cup of skim milk, for instance, provides 300 milligrams of calcium, as well as supplemental vitamin D. But to be on the safe side, take 1,500 milligrams in supplement form a day.

Look to Lubricants

✐ Vaginal dryness, the result of waning estrogen levels, may dampen your interest in sex. Try a **water-soluble lubricant**, such as Astroglide or K-Y Silky. Avoid oil-based lubricants such as petroleum jelly. Studies suggest that the oil-based kind don't work as well and can actually increase irritation if used long-term.

Skip it!

Some women turn to progesterone creams or suppositories to ease menopause symptoms. But doctors and researchers are concerned that overuse of progesterone might raise the risk of breast cancer. Talk to your doctor before using the cream.

Menstrual Problems

Long ago, people used to believe that the presence of a menstruating woman could turn milk sour and make meat go bad. Beliefs have changed—now the assumption is that menstruation turns moods sour and makes tempers go bad. Preconceptions aside, there are ways to make the cycles easier. When you need quick relief from cramps or lower-back pain, ibuprofen (the active ingredient in Advil and Motrin) can help. In addition, there are many other ways to find relief and—with patience and foresight—prevent next month's discomfort.

What's wrong

Cramps, bloating, backache, nausea, headache, and fatigue—any or all of these menstrual problems can result from hormonal fluctuations in a woman's monthly cycle. Some of them are related to prostaglandins, hormone-like substances that cause the muscles in the uterus to tighten, leading to cramping. During the 7 to 10 days before your period, there's also a drop in production of the hormone progesterone, which causes your body to retain salt and water. And an imbalance between progesterone and the hormone estrogen contributes to emotional symptoms such as depression, anxiety, and irritability.

Take Anti-Cramp Action

When you feel cramps coming on, go for a walk or run. Or jump in the pool for a swim. Or get on an exercise bike. Any kind of **exercise** (including sex!) helps inhibit prostaglandin production and boosts the release of painkilling endorphins. As a bonus, exercise can also help relieve bloating.

Soak in a tub of **hot water**. The warmth helps relax knotted-up muscles in the uterus. Or lie down with a hot-water bottle or heating pad on your abdomen.

Try a homeopathic remedy. For severe cramps, experts recommend **mag phos** (phosphate of magnesia). Take five pellets of 6C or 12C every hour for five doses. If the cramps don't improve, take the same dosage of **nux vomica** or **pulsitilla**. Nux vomica is usually recommended for cramps that are accompanied by constipation and extreme irritability, and pulsitilla is advised when you find yourself not only cramping, but weeping as well.

Tame Cramps with Tea

During the day, have three cups of warm **red raspberry-leaf tea**. (Look for raspberry-leaf tea bags at the grocery store or a health-food store.) Raspberry leaves contain fragrine, a substance that tones the uterus and helps ease cramping. It can also lighten excessive bleeding.

As its name implies, **cramp bark** (*Viburnum opulus*) can

take the edge off cramps. Buy the dried bark and make a tea using 1 teaspoon bark in 1 cup water, or buy the tincture and follow the dosage directions on the label.

🌿 Good old **chamomile tea** has antispasmodic properties to unclench your uterus. Use 2 to 4 teaspoons of herb per cup of hot water, or buy chamomile tea bags. Peppermint is another antispasmodic herb.

🌿 **Ginger** is another tried-and-true cramp remedy. It's thought to work by inhibiting the production of prostaglandins. To make the tea, grate 1 teaspoon fresh gingerroot, add 1 cup hot water, steep for 10 minutes, then strain.

Beat the Bloat

🌿 To deal with bloating, **reduce the salt** in your diet and take **vitamin B$_6$** during your period. During the week before your period, use the saltshaker as little as possible and also cut back on other high-sodium foods, such as packaged meats, canned soups, and salty snacks. Meanwhile, take 25 to 50 milligrams of vitamin B$_6$ every day. This vitamin appears to have a mild diuretic effect.

Manage the Flow

🌿 Every day take 1,000 milligrams of **vitamin C** and 1,000 milligrams of **bioflavonoids** in divided doses—500 milligrams of each in the morning, then another 500 milligrams in the evening. Both supplements help strengthen the walls of the blood vessels to reduce excessive bleeding. Bioflavonoids are found in grape skins, blackberries, blueberries, and citrus fruits, especially in the pulp and white rind.

🌿 **Chaste tree**, typically used as a PMS remedy, also helps regulate the menstrual cycle by balancing levels of sex hormones. (In men it can lower libido, so in days of old it was fed to priests, hence the name chasteberry.) Try it to lighten a heavy flow. The dosage is 40 drops (in tincture form) or 225 milligrams (in capsule form) a day.

The Power of Prevention

🌿 Every day take 1,000 milligrams of **calcium citrate**. Calcium is a natural tonic and muscle relaxer. It helps to reduce

Should I call **the doctor?**

Give your doctor a call if your cycles are shorter than 21 days, or if you go more than 35 days between menstrual periods. You'll also want to contact the doctor if you bleed heavily for more than a week, quickly soaking through your tampons or pads, or if you pass large clots of blood. (Small clots, no larger than the size of a quarter, are normal.) And the doctor might help if you experience severe cramps that over-the-counter medication can't relieve.

the ferocity of menstrual cramping. (Avoid coral-derived calcium, as it is subject to contamination with heavy metals.)

⟿ Take 200 milligrams of **elemental magnesium** two or three times a day. The supplements come in the form of magnesium glycinate, magnesium citrate, and magnesium oxide. All help prevent menstrual cramps, but the citrate and oxide forms also have a laxative effect. Use glycinate if you don't need to worry about regularity.

⟿ Essential fatty acids slow the production of prostaglandins, which contribute to cramps. Get your fill by taking 1,000 milligrams of **evening primrose oil** three times a day or 1 tablespoon of **flaxseed oil** a day (use it in salad dressings in place of other oils).

⟿ During the last 2 weeks of your cycle, take 15 drops of **black cohosh** in tincture form three times a day. This herb is an antispasmodic, which means it relaxes the uterus and reduces cramping.

Muscle Cramps

Something as simple as heat or massage can strong-hand cramps into submission. Once the agony is over, it's important to mount an anti-cramp campaign. Your body is probably yearning for potassium, magnesium, and calcium—the trio of minerals that helps regulate activity in your nerves and muscles. (You have potassium aplenty if you eat fruits and veggies, but you may be potassium poor if you're on a high-protein diet.) You'll also need to drink plenty of water and stretch your limits regularly.

Put the Heat On

Place an electric **heating pad** or a **hot washcloth** on the misbehaving muscle to relax the cramp and increase blood flow to the affected tissue. Set the pad on low, apply for 20 minutes, then remove it for at least 20 minutes before reapplying.

Take a long, warm shower, or soak in the bath. For added relief, pour in a half-cup **Epsom salt**. The magnesium in Epsom salt promotes muscle relaxation.

Press Out Pain

Find the epicenter of the cramp. Press into this spot with your thumb, the heel of your hand, or a loosely clenched fist. Hold the pressure for 10 seconds, ease up for 10 seconds, then press again. You're doing it right if you feel some discomfort, but not excruciating pain. After a number of repetitions, the pain from the cramp should start to diminish.

Rub It In

Mix 1 part **wintergreen oil** with 4 parts **vegetable oil**, and massage it into the cramp. Wintergreen contains methyl salicylate (related to aspirin), which relieves pain and stimulates blood flow. You can use this mixture several times a day, but not with a heating pad—you could burn your skin.

Banish Nighttime Leg Cramps

Before bed, drink a glass of **tonic water**, which contains quinine, a popular remedy for leg cramps. Research has sup-

What's **wrong**

Sometimes you get a cramp during a workout. But it can also happen after some part of your body has remained frozen in one position for hours—say, gripping a pen or a paintbrush. In either case, the cramps are caused by overuse of a muscle, dehydration, stress, or fatigue. But if calves cramp painfully when you're trying to sleep, or a muscle often locks up for no apparent reason, the root cause is a faulty chemical signal from the nervous system that "tells" the muscle to contract. Often the problem is linked to an imbalance of potassium and sodium.

Should I call the doctor?

Muscle cramps are usually temporary and don't cause permanent damage. But give your doctor a call if the cramp or spasm lasts for more than a day, or if it continues to bother you despite trying home remedies. And call immediately if the spasm occurs in the lower back or neck and is accompanied by pain that radiates down your leg or into your arm, or if abdominal cramps occur in the lower-right-hand part of your belly, which could signal appendicitis.

ported the use of quinine for nocturnal leg cramps, but **don't take quinine tablets**; they can have serious side effects, such as ringing in the ears and disturbed vision. The FDA has banned the sale of the tablets.

To prevent nighttime calf cramps, **try not to sleep with your toes pointed**. And don't tuck in your sheets too tightly—this tends to bend your toes downward, activating cramps.

Take 400 to 800 IU of **vitamin E** to prevent nocturnal leg cramps. Studies suggest that taking vitamin E improves blood flow through the arteries.

Mind Your Minerals

Low levels of minerals known as electrolytes—which include potassium, sodium, calcium, and magnesium—can contribute to cramps. You probably don't need any more sodium in your diet, but you may need more of the others. Good food sources of **magnesium** are whole-grain breads and cereals, nuts, and beans. You can get **potassium** from most fruits and vegetables, especially bananas, oranges, and cantaloupes. And dairy foods supply **calcium**.

If you change your diet and you still get cramps, take 500 milligrams of **calcium** and 500 milligrams of **magnesium** twice a day, for a total of 1,000 milligrams of each supplement. Some people who get leg cramps due to a magnesium deficiency find fast relief from taking supplements. Don't take magnesium without calcium; the two minerals work as a pair.

Taking a diuretic for high blood pressure? Your increased need to urinate may be robbing you of potassium. The result: a condition called **hypokalemia**, which can cause fatigue, muscle weakness, and muscle cramps. Ask your doctor if you can switch to a blood-pressure medication that isn't a diuretic.

Drink Your Fill

Cramps are often caused by dehydration, so if you're getting frequent cramps, drink more **water**.

If you tend to get cramps during exercise, drink at least 2 cups of water two hours before each workout. Then stop and drink 4 to 8 ounces every 10 to 20 minutes during your exercise sessions. If you're sweating a lot, consider a **sports drink**, such as Gatorade, that replaces lost sodium and other electrolytes.

Nail Problems

There are people who really care for their nails, while others couldn't care less. Whether or not you're the manicure type, though, you'll want to seek some help when fingernails or toenails turn into eyesores. Here are some ways to get them back in shape fast with better nutrition, selected supplements, and fungus-fighters.

Foil Fungus

 To fight stubborn nail fungus, try **tea-tree oil**. A powerful antiseptic, it can help make nail fungus disappear. In fact, in one study it proved to be as effective as a prescription antifungal medicine. Once or twice a day, apply a drop or two to the discolored nail. A good time to do it is after you bathe or shower, when your skin is softest.

 Alternatively, you can use an **antifungal powder** that absorbs moisture and prevents fungus. Some good ones are Zeasorb-AF powder or Ammens Medicated Powder. You can sprinkle a medicated antifungal powder into your socks too.

 If your feet are sweaty when you get home, change into a **fresh pair of socks** right away. And if you have an office job, take along a pair of clean socks—especially on hot summer days—so you can change before you start work.

 Don't clip your cuticles. When you do this, you're removing your nail's protective barrier. Fungi and bacteria find it easier to get a grip around the base of the nail after the cuticle is removed.

Say No to Weak Nails

 Take 300 micrograms of **biotin**, a B vitamin, 4 to 6 times a day with food. Long ago, veterinarians learned that this vitamin could strengthen horses' hooves—and the hooves are made primarily from keratin, the same material that makes up human nails. If your nails are weak or brittle, biotin might be all you need to strengthen and thicken them. But it doesn't

What's **wrong**

Apart from ingrown toenails, nail fungus is probably the most disagreeable nail problem. When you get this affliction—usually on a toenail—the nail turns thick, discolored, and crumbly. Other nail problems include brittle nails, which can be the result of age or too much or too little moisture, or nutritional deficiencies. And certain skin diseases can affect the nails, including psoriasis (it can cause a thickening and pitting of the nails) and the patchy hair loss known as alopecia areata (it can cause ridged, pitted, rough nails).

Should I call **the doctor?**

Unless you suspect you have an underlying nutritional deficiency, brittle nails are cosmetic issues rather than health issues. As for nail fungus, it's tenacious, and it can take months—or years—to clear up on its own, so ask a doctor if you might benefit from prescription medication.

work right away. You'll need to take this treatment for six months or more before you see a noticeable difference.

 Drink a cup of **horsetail** or **nettle tea** once a day. These herbs are high in silica and other minerals that nails need to grow.

Eat for Beautiful Nails

 If your nails are brittle or flaking, try getting more essential fatty acids. These are found in foods such as **fatty fish** and **flaxseed** or **flaxseed oil**. If you don't eat much fish, take 1 tablespoon flaxseed oil a day (use it in place of other oil in salad dressing), or sprinkle ground flaxseeds on your cereal or other food.

 Evening primrose oil is another source of essential fatty acid. Take 1,000 milligrams three times a day with meals.

 If your nails have white spots, you may be deficient in **zinc**. Nuts, root vegetables, whole grains, meat, and shellfish are good sources of this mineral.

Moisturize and Protect

 For dry, brittle nails, rub **petroleum jelly** or a thick cream into your nails to hold moisture around and under your nails. If you do this at bedtime, slip a pair of thin cotton gloves on your hands before you go to sleep.

 Wear **vinyl gloves** every time you wash dishes or do other household tasks that require you to immerse your hands in water. (Vinyl is best, because people with nail problems tend to have skin that is sensitive to rubber.)

 Avoid polish removers that contain acetone or formaldehyde. They're terribly drying to nails. Use **acetate-based** removers instead.

Fake Nails Breed Fungus

For women who have problems with weak, soft, brittle nails, artificial nails can seem like a godsend. But if you want to avoid nail fungus, forgo the fakes, no matter how much you long for elegant nails. Artificial nails are glued on top of your real ones, and the gap in-between creates a breeding ground for fungus. Even worse, this is an area where you can develop a painful bacterial infection. Artificial nails are the most common cause of nail fungus in women.

Nausea

When nausea tells you that something inside your stomach wants to get out, doctors agree that you shouldn't try to induce vomiting. But if it's going to happen naturally, then go ahead and let it. If you have a milder case of queasiness, try these tummy tamers to get your stomach feeling like it's back on dry land instead of tossing on stormy seas.

Teas for the Queasy

🌿 One of the oldest and perhaps the best remedies is ginger, proven to allay both nausea and motion sickness. Try a warm cup of **ginger tea**. Peel away the root bark, then chop or grate the whitish part of the root until you have one full teaspoon. Put the gratings in a mug, add a cup of boiling water, cover with a saucer, and let it steep for 10 minutes. You can drink the tea when it's still warm or after it has cooled down a bit. If you don't have any fresh gingerroot, try eating a few gingersnaps or a piece of crystallized ginger.

🌿 Second to ginger is **peppermint**, which has a calming effect on the lining of the stomach. There are many brands of peppermint tea, sold in bags or loose-tea form, and you can drink a cup anytime you feel nauseous.

Sip Sweet Stuff

🌿 Drinks containing sugar are likely to calm a shaky stomach. One recommendation is **cola syrup**, which can be found in some pharmacies. If your drugstore doesn't have it, just open a bottle of cola and let it go flat, shaking it every once in a while to dispel the fizz. Drink it at room temperature.

🌿 Some people get great results with flat **7-Up** or **ginger ale**.

🌿 Create a homemade **anti-nausea syrup**. Put a half-cup white sugar and a quarter-cup water into a saucepan, turn the heat to medium, and stir steadily until you have a clear syrup. After the syrup cools to room temperature, take 1 to 2 tablespoons as needed.

What's **wrong**

Nausea happens when the nausea and vomiting center in the brain stem is activated. It can be caused by motion sickness, morning sickness that accompanies pregnancy, and the stomach flu. Sometimes it's a natural reaction to something you've eaten—something bad the body wants to get rid of. A concussion, heart attack, some types of cancer, and chemotherapy can also trigger nausea. So can prescription drugs and OTC medications.

If nausea leads to vomiting, you may lose a lot of salts and fluids. To recover—and avoid dehydration—you need to replace what you've lost. One way is to make a rehydration drink by dissolving 8 level teaspoons sugar and 1 teaspoon salt in 1 quart water. Drink small sips to start, then more as your stomach settles down. Alternatively, a sports drink such as Gatorade will do the trick.

Should I call **the doctor?**

If you've been queasy for several days, tell your doctor. And be sure to call the doctor if you start to vomit profusely, if the vomit is bloody, if you've been unable to keep food or liquids down for 24 hours, or if you've taken a bad fall or had a severe blow to the head. Heart attacks are sometimes accompanied by nausea, so call immediately if your nausea is accompanied by severe, sudden chest pain.

Be Still

When you're nauseated, **lie still**. Moving around disturbs the balance mechanism in your middle ear, which can worsen nausea and lead to vomiting. While you're lying down, place a cool washcloth on your forehead and focus on your breathing so you don't think as much about your stomach.

Press the Anti-Nausea Point

Try this **acupressure** trick: Place your right thumb on the inside of your left forearm, about two thumb-widths from the crease of your wrist. Press firmly for about a minute, then move your thumb a little closer to your wrist and press for another minute. Repeat on the other forearm.

Calm with Carbs

If you're hungry (despite the nausea) and you think you can handle it, eat some **toast** or a few **crackers**, foods that are high in carbohydrates. As your stomach starts to calm down, add a bit of light protein—cooked chicken breast, for instance. But don't eat foods that contain fat until you're feeling a lot better.

Nosebleed

They tend to occur at the most inopportune moments, and the sudden gushing of blood from your face can be both embarrassing and frightening, especially since a small amount can seem like gallons when it's soaking tissue after tissue with crimson. Don't panic. Usually you can halt a nosebleed—and save face—in a matter of minutes. Here are some effective ways to do it.

Pinch, Press, and Spray

➤ The simplest remedy for a bloody nose is the time-honored **pinch cure**. Sit up straight with your head tilted slightly forward (to keep the blood from running down your throat). Gently blow out any clots that could prevent a vessel from sealing. Then pinch the soft part of your nose and press firmly toward your face. Hold that position for at least 10 minutes.

➤ Tired of pinching? Use a **clothespin**.

➤ Still dripping? Wad up a small piece of **tissue** or **gauze**, then stick it between your gums and upper lip in the area right under your nose. Leave it there for 5 to 10 minutes. The tissue puts pressure on the blood vessels that are sending blood to your nose. There are countless versions of this remedy—pouring vinegar, witch hazel, or lemon juice on the tissue; using a small square of brown paper from a bag sprinkled with salt; even placing a dime or a small, flat button under your upper lip instead of a tissue.

➤ Apply an **ice pack** alongside the bleeding nostril. The cold narrows the blood vessels in the nose to slow the spurting.

➤ If your nose still doesn't stop dripping, sniff some **nasal spray**, such as Afrin or Neo-Synephrine. Like ice, it will constrict the vessels in your nose, stanching the flow of blood.

The Power of Prevention

➤ If you want to avoid nosebleeds, keep your mucous membranes moist by drinking eight 8-ounce glasses of water a day. You are well hydrated if your urine is pale, not dark.

What's **wrong**

Maybe you ran into a door or blew your nose too hard. Now your nose is leaking—or pouring—blood. Regardless of the precipitating factor, a nosebleed occurs when blood vessels rupture inside a nostril. Often, that happens when the sensitive inner lining of the nose becomes irritated by dry indoor heat or air conditioning. People with high blood pressure or hardening of the arteries (atherosclerosis) are particularly vulnerable to bloody noses, along with those who take certain medications, including anti-inflammatory drugs such as aspirin or ibuprofen or blood thinners such as warfarin (Coumadin).

Should I call
the doctor?

Call your doctor if your nosebleed is the result of a blow to the head, especially if the blood appears thin and watery (it suggests the presence of cerebral fluid). Also call if the nosebleed doesn't stop within 30 minutes, if you feel weak or faint, or if your nose bleeds frequently for no apparent reason. Anyone who has been diagnosed with high blood pressure should call his doctor if a nosebleed continues for more than 10 minutes.

Don't overdo the AC. Air-conditioning dries out the air, leaving you more prone to nosebleeds.

In winter, add moisture indoors by running a **humidifier**.

Dab the insides of your nose with **petroleum jelly**, or spritz your nostrils liberally with a **saline nasal spray**. Either method will help keep nostrils moist. This approach is helpful if you're about to take a plane flight, if you've just recovered from a cold or sinus infection, or if you live in a very dry climate.

Watch your aspirin intake. Aspirin can interfere with blood clotting, and of course that's not a good thing if you get frequent nosebleeds.

If you have **nasal allergies**, treat them promptly. Between the constant irritation caused by allergens and the damage done by blowing your nose, nasal membranes take a real beating when you're having an allergic reaction.

If you often have trouble with nosebleeds, take 1,000 to 1,200 milligrams of **vitamin C** every day to help prevent them. Vitamin C helps strengthen capillary walls and is also a vital component of collagen, a substance that gives your nostrils a moist, protective lining. Along with vitamin C, take 500 milligrams daily of a **bioflavonoid supplement** such as grape-seed extract, pine-bark extract, pycnogenol, or proanthocyanins. Flavonoids are known to heal capillaries.

Poison Ivy

No one would knowingly touch a toxic plant, yet generations of even sharp-eyed outdoors people, not to mention kids wandering in the woods, have picked up the itch. If you know you've been exposed, you may be able to wash off the allergy-inducing urushiol before it's too late. And there are many ways to ease the itching and dry the blisters if you do get poison ivy. But avoidance is by far the best approach—especially if you're one of those people driven nuts by itching.

Rush to Wash

➤ Run for the shower—or the nearest creek, if you're hiking—and **wash away the resin** before the allergic reaction takes hold. Once you come into contact with poison ivy, the clock starts ticking: You have about 15 minutes to get rid of the urushiol. Use soap and warm water, if they're available. If you have a choice of soaps, use one that does not contain moisturizers. Skip the washcloth, since it can spread the oil around your body.

➤ If it's impossible to wash right away, clean your skin with **rubbing alcohol** to dissolve the urushiol. If none is handy, you can use any product (or beverage) that contains alcohol.

➤ Alternatively, you can clean off the urushiol with **Tecnu**, an over-the-counter solvent that's designed especially to remove urushiol from the skin. Tecnu is very effective at removing the resin, but be sure to rinse it off immediately or you risk skin irritation.

A Gem of a Cure

➤ If you know what the **jewelweed** plant looks like (it has tall, translucent stems and hanging, trumpet-shaped yellow or orange flowers) and there's one growing nearby, crush a handful of the leaves and stems and smear the juice on the affected area. Also known as impatiens and touch-me-not, this plant sometimes grows near poison ivy. There is some research to support the old folk notion that it works against poison ivy rash.

What's wrong

Seven out of ten people are allergic to poison ivy, making this the world's most common allergy. People who have the allergy are sensitive to urushiol, an irritating resin that's found in poison ivy, poison oak, and poison sumac. If you so much as brush one of these plants, urushiol can get on your skin. Within as little as two hours, you'll develop an itchy rash that will have you scratching for three weeks or more. You can also get the rash by touching clothes or other items that have been contaminated with urushiol. And if there's urushiol on your fingers, you'll be spreading the rash around your body every time you scratch.

Should I call **the doctor?**

If you're in extreme discomfort, or if you have severe blistering, swelling, or redness, call your doctor. You should also alert the doctor if you might have inhaled the smoke of burning poison ivy plants, particularly if you become short of breath. Seek medical attention at once if the rash is on your eyes, nose, mouth, throat, or genitals.

Other Plant Remedies

Slice a leaf of a fresh **aloe vera** plant, scoop out the gel, and apply to the affected areas. Aloe is not only for sunburn; its anti-inflammatory and antibacterial properties make it great for poison ivy as well. Commercial aloe vera gel products are fine if they are made mostly from pure gel from the plant.

Pick a few leaves from the common lawn weed **plantain,** wash them, mash them, and apply as a poultice to the affected skin. Plantain contains a chemical (called allantoin) that is anti-inflammatory and antimicrobial.

Stop the Spread

Wash the clothes you were wearing when you touched poison ivy in the washing machine with warm water. This should get out all the urushiol so the rash won't spread.

Rinse off your shoes. If you were wearing washable sneakers when you came into contact with the plant, put them through a separate cycle after washing your clothes.

Dogs and cats don't get poison ivy, but their **fur** can become coated with urushiol. So if Fido followed you into the woods, you can either avoid him for the next few days or give him a bath in soapy water. The bath is a real chore, however, since you'll have to wear rubber gloves and a raincoat to avoid getting urushiol on your skin.

Attack the Itch

Use a **vinegar** compress to dry the rash and relieve itching. Mix a half-cup white vinegar with 1½ cups water. Chill in the refrigerator. When you need cool relief, moisten a cloth in the solution and press it onto the rash.

Dab **calamine lotion** onto the rash. This classic poison ivy remedy relieves itch and will help dry up blisters. If you find the lotion too runny, just mix in a little **cornstarch**.

Soak a cloth in **cold milk** and hold it against your skin. Cold milk is more soothing to itchy skin than cold water. Exactly why milk relieves itching is unknown, but perhaps it's the milk fat.

Using a cotton ball, treat your rash with **witch hazel**, which has a great reputation as a skin soother. The kind that comes in an alcohol solution cools your skin as it evaporates.

- Moisten a plain old **tea bag** (black or green, it doesn't matter) and apply it to the itchy skin. The tannic acid in tea, which is astringent, helps contract inflamed tissue and relieve the itching.

- Take a warm bath to which you've added a few table-spoons of **colloidal oatmeal** (like Aveeno) or plain oatmeal ground in a blender. The oatmeal will help dry a rash that has started to blister, and also relieves the itch. Be careful when getting out—oatmeal makes the tub very slippery.

- To dry out the rash, relax in a bath containing **Epsom salt**. Follow the label directions.

The Power of Prevention

- Whenever venturing out into the wilds where you may come into contact with poisonous plants, wear **long pants** and a **long-sleeved shirt**.

- Get a plant-identification book, and **learn to recognize poison ivy, oak, and sumac.** Many people recognize poison ivy for its "leaves of three." But they may fail to recognize that poison ivy can grow as a shrub or tree-clinging vine as well as a ground cover. In the spring, its leaves are reddish. Late in the season, it bears pale white berries.

- Before going out, rub some **IvyBlock** or **Stokogard** out-door cream on exposed skin. These claylike lotions, which are available over the counter, form a protective barrier that guards skin against urushiol.

- **Don't go near any burning brush pile**. If there's poison ivy in the pile, the oil takes to the air and can get into your lungs. You can develop a serious lung infection, as well as a rash over your entire body.

Tried...

Before there was calamine lotion, people used white shoe polish on poison ivy rash.

...and true

Shoe polish in the old-fashioned shake-up bottle contains pipe clay, which is similar to one of the main ingredients in calamine.

Old **wives' tale**

Poison ivy blisters sometimes become filled with fluid, and some people think that the fluid spreads the rash. Not true. It's harmless. Only oil from the plant can cause the rash.

Prostate Enlargement

Here's another example why "aging gracefully" is an oxymoron. After years of doing bathroom business with due dispatch, many a male turns grim-faced when the usual stance turns unproductive. First? Check your medicine cabinet for OTCs such as antihistamines and decongestants that might be making the problem worse. Then, after you've cleared out those troublemakers, try some supplements and check your diet. For the male in a bind, many of these remedies, used alone or in combination, can make the trouble far more tolerable.

What's wrong

After age 40, many men start to notice that their personal plumbing isn't working properly. Urine comes out with difficulty, the flow is weak, and urination ends with dribbles. Most irritating of all, nature calls during the night, and sleep suffers. The cause is often benign prostatic hyperplasia (BPH). This is a noncancerous swelling of the prostate, the gland that produces seminal fluid. Since the prostate surrounds the urethra—the tube running from the bladder out through the penis—when that gland swells, it blocks the flow of urine. After age 60, at least half of all men have some degree of prostate swelling.

Gladden Your Gland with Herbs

🌿 Take 160 milligrams of **saw palmetto** in capsule form twice daily. Look for an extract containing 85% to 95% fatty acids and sterols. This supplement, which contains extracts of the berries of the saw palmetto plant, seems to block the action of a hormone called dihydrotestosterone, which stimulates growth in the prostate gland. There is evidence that it also decreases inflammation.

🌿 Twice a day, take 50 to 200 milligrams of **pygeum africanum**, a supplement that comes from the bark of an African tree. Like saw palmetto, it has a long history of relieving benign prostatic hyperplasia (BPH), apparently by interfering with dihydrotestosterone.

🌿 You may find that taking a supplement containing **both saw palmetto and pygeum** works better than taking either of the herbs alone. If you go this route, look for a brand containing about 320 milligrams of saw palmetto and about 100 milligrams of pygeum.

🌿 Look for supplements containing extract of dried **nettle root** extract and take 200 to 400 milligrams in capsule form three times a day. Nettle root helps shrink the prostate, and when taken with pygeum, it seems to help that supplement work better.

🌿 The antioxidant **lycopene** decreases inflammation and swelling of the prostate gland. The effective dose is 10 to 20 milligrams daily, taken in combination with other supplements that help control BPH. A number of brand-name supplements such as ProstaThera include lycopene along with a combination of other BPH relievers such as serenoa, pygeum, urtica, and zinc chelate.

Give Your Prostate the Food It Needs

🔹 Eat a handful of unroasted **pumpkin seeds** each day. The seeds, which are an old folk remedy for prostate enlargement still often recommended today, are a rich source of zinc.

🔹 Eat lots of **tomatoes** or tomato-based products—as many as 10 servings per week. Tomatoes are rich in lycopene, the prostate-friendly antioxidant described above. **Watermelon** and **apricots** also are rich in lycopene.

🔹 Twice a day, mix a tablespoon of **flaxseed oil** in your food. It is a rich source of omega-3 fatty acids. These and other essential fatty acids decrease inflammation in the prostate gland (and thus reduce swelling) by limiting the concentration of the hormone prostaglandin.

Be a Picky Drinker

🔹 Cut back on fluids in the evening, as you'll more likely have to get up in the night. You need plenty of fluids, but **drink before dinnertime**, not after.

🔹 If you're already having trouble urinating, **limit** the number of caffeinated drinks you consume, such as **coffee, tea**, and **sodas**. Caffeine tends to make the outlet from your bladder tighten, creating a roadblock that interferes with urine flow. It's also a diuretic, which is exactly what you don't want if you're already getting up to urinate during the night.

🔹 Also **cut back on alcohol**—or, better yet, forgo it completely. Like caffeine, it causes constriction at the neck of the bladder, and acts as a diuretic.

Keep Your Prostate Running on Empty

🔹 **Ejaculate regularly**, either through intercourse or alone. The prostate gland produces the nutrient-rich fluid in which the sperm are bathed, and ejaculation helps to relieve the internal fluid pressure. It also helps keep the gland from becoming inflamed.

Should I call **the doctor?**

When you have trouble starting to urinate, a weak urine stream, a feeling that your bladder can't totally empty, and a frequent need to go during the night, you should have a checkup. The doctor can tell whether you have BPH and rule out other conditions, particularly prostate cancer. More severe symptoms call for an emergency room visit. If you can't urinate, even with straining, for more than 8 hours, this is urinary obstruction. You need immediate treatment to prevent kidney failure.

Tried...

Some men say you should get up and walk around as much as possible to help deal with a problem prostate.

...and true

When you remain sitting, you put pressure on your prostate. In fact, men who sit for long periods while they work—such as truck drivers—report more BPH than those who are frequently moving around. If you have a desk job, get up and pace every once in a while.

Lounge in the Tub

Sit in **warm water**. The heat will increase blood flow in the prostate gland, which helps reduce swelling and inflammation. If you can, spend 20 to 45 minutes in the tub every day.

Let It Flow

Urinate **whenever you get the urge.** Some men seem to think it's best to exercise bladder control and avoid trips to the bathroom. But when the bladder is too full, urine gets into the prostate, irritating it.

When in the bathroom, **urinate as much as possible,** relax for a few minutes, and then urinate again. Doctors call this "double voiding." It's a good way to guarantee that you have emptied your bladder completely.

Try sitting on the toilet to urinate rather than standing. The combination of the new position and the more relaxed situation can make for a more effective bathroom visit.

Relax in the bathroom. This is not a contest, no one is judging, no one is timing you. Read something, ponder something, take 10 slow, deep breaths in a row. Why? Tension and anxiety trigger stress hormones that can cause the bladder muscles to tense up. If you are putting too much psychological pressure on yourself to "perform," that alone can stop the performance. No reason to turn a physical problem into a psychological one as well.

Psoriasis

There are good days and there are bad days, and if you're troubled with psoriasis, you know the difference all too well. On the good days, you hardly need to pay attention to what your skin's doing. On the bad ones, red itchy patches are crying for attention. Here are ways to make good days better and the bad more bearable.

See the Light

🔹 **Sunlight** is an excellent remedy for psoriasis. Every day, spend 15 to 30 minutes in the sun, and you should see results in less than six weeks. While doctors don't have the full explanation, research shows that sunlight decreases the activity of the skin's T cells. These specialized cells produce substances called cytokines, which initiate a cycle of inflammation. When you expose T cells to sunlight, it quells their action, breaking the cycle.

🔹 Protect yourself from burning by wearing **sunscreen** with an SPF of at least 15 on healthy areas of skin.

Go Skin Dipping

🔹 Take a good, long soak in warm water . . . then add some **vegetable oil**. Here's why: A long bath can soften scaly patches and soothe itching, but bathing can also dry your skin and make itching worse. So sit in the tub for about 10 minutes, letting your skin get thoroughly soaked, but about 5 minutes before you get out, add a few spoonfuls of vegetable oil. That's all it takes to seal the water into your skin. (Be careful getting out of the tub, because oil makes the tub slippery.)

🔹 To relieve itching, try a cool-water bath, adding **vinegar** to the bathwater. Many people find that vinegar helps psoriasis, even though doctors aren't sure why. What's known is that acetic acid in vinegar kills bacteria—and one theory holds that psoriasis is made worse by bacteria.

🔹 Fine-ground **oatmeal** is another good ingredient for itch relief. You can sprinkle in an oatmeal product specially made

What's wrong

Your skin is growing too fast. Normally, new skin cells need about 28 days to migrate from deep within your skin to the surface, where they replace dead cells that fall away. But if you have psoriasis, the cycle is compressed into about four days. Skin cells pile up, causing distinctive red, bumpy patches covered with white scales. These frequently develop on the knees, elbows, and scalp. The cause is unknown, but psoriasis seems to be more prevalent in some families than in others. People with psoriasis tend to have flare-ups, when the rashes get worse, followed by intervals when the condition is far less severe.

Should I call **the doctor?**

If an outbreak covers a wide area of skin, or affects the palms of your hands and soles of your feet, you'll want to see the doctor. You also need a doctor's attention whenever you see signs of infection, such as pus or a yellow crust on your skin. If your psoriasis is accompanied by joint pain, a condition called psoriatic arthritis, you need to be under a doctor's care. And if you develop widespread bumps containing pus and have a fever, it's an emergency: Call a doctor to deal with the infection immediately.

for bathing, such as Aveeno. Or put unflavored oatmeal in a blender, grind it until it turns into a fine powder, then sprinkle it in the water.

Don Another Layer

After bathing, spread on a moisturizing cream to lock in your skin's natural moisture. Make sure to add a thick layer to the psoriasis patches. This helps prevent cracking. Avoid liquid lotions, which dry up too quickly, and instead choose a heavy cream or ointment. Among the best are **Lacticare** or **Amlactin**, which contain lactic acid to prevent skin from drying out, or **Carmol** cream, which contains urea to help loosen scales.

Try **Bag Balm**, a product originally designed for use on cows' udders. It's gained a reputation for soothing dry, cracked skin. Look for it in farm-supply stores or pharmacies.

Try a cream that contains **chamomile**, if you can find one. This plant has a long-held reputation for reducing inflammation and soothing flaky skin.

Rub a few drops of **tea-tree oil** into your psoriasis patches several times a day. This Australian remedy is useful for relieving itch and softening psoriasis patches, especially if you have a mild case. However, some people have an allergic reaction to tea-tree oil, so be sure to test on a small patch of skin. Also, the skin covered with tea-tree oil may have increased sensitivity to sunlight.

To soften the skin and remove scaly patches, you can also use **petroleum jelly**. Apply it as often as necessary.

Get Oiled

Mix a tablespoon of **flaxseed oil** into your cereal, yogurt, or other food each day. This isn't for flavoring—it's for your psoriasis. Flaxseed oil is high in omega-3 fatty acids, and these compounds help to block a chemical in your body called arachidonic acid, which causes inflammation.

Oily fish are also high in omega-3s. If you like **salmon**, it's a good idea to have it at least once a week. Other fish that are high in omega-3s are **sardines** and **mackerel**.

You can also get these fatty acids by taking 1,000 milligrams of **fish oil** three times a day. Large amounts of fish oil can "thin" the blood, so check with your doctor first if you're taking a blood thinner such as aspirin or coumadin.

~ If you have an **aloe vera** plant on your shelf, break a stem and apply the gel several times a day to itchy patches of skin. Aloe has anti-inflammatory compounds, and the gel contains magnesium lactate, which helps control itching.

Avoid Getting into Scrapes

~ **Keep your hands off** the red spots. Even minor damage to your skin can worsen your psoriasis symptoms. If you pick and scratch the itchy patches, you'll damage your skin, which can lead to more extensive outbreaks.

~ Always use an **electric shaver** instead of a razor if you have psoriasis on your legs, face, or other areas where you shave. A sharp razor nicks your skin, no matter how careful you are, which raises your risk of new outbreaks. Shavers are gentler.

The Ticket to Scalp Care

~ If you get psoriasis on your scalp, it's time to shop for special shampoos. You want a product that contains **salicylic acid** or **tar**. Effective shampoos (with 2% tar) include Neutrogena T/Gel Extra Strength or DHS Tar. Use daily at first, then twice a week—alternating with regular shampoo—as symptoms subside. When you apply the shampoo, leave it in contact with your scalp for 10 minutes before rinsing.

~ Keep a list of several shampoos that you like. Whenever you finish one kind, rotate and choose another. Your scalp may become tolerant to one kind of shampoo that becomes less effective if you use it long-term. People report better results if they **switch shampoos**.

~ Adopt a **short hairstyle**. With a simple do, it will be a lot easier to treat your scalp.

Simmer Down

~ Get regular **exercise**. It's a great stress reducer—and stress is known to contribute to outbreaks. If you can take a 30-minute walk every day, you may be surprised at how effectively that token amount of exercise distracts you from things that are getting you keyed up.

~ Practice a relaxing mental exercise, such as **meditating** or **deep breathing**, a few minutes each day.

Did you **know?**

For reasons that are not well understood, cold temperatures aggravate psoriasis. You can't change the seasons, of course, but you might be able to keep outbreaks in check if you dress warmly and keep your skin well covered when you're out in the cold.

Skip it!

Sunlight is helpful for treating psoriasis, but stay away from tanning booths. The artificial light doesn't cover the same spectrum as sunlight, and won't help your condition.

Restless Legs Syndrome

Of all our body's mysteries, this is surely among the quirkiest. When you're otherwise ready for rest, why should your legs keep running? When every fiber of your being says, "Settle down!" why are you gamely kicking your bedmate? Since RLS seems to be related to mineral imbalances, perhaps the best place to end the night race is with supplements. But if they don't stop your in-place pacing, you'll want to develop some pre-bed rituals to help those legs settle down.

What's wrong

The name restless legs syndrome (RLS) pretty much describes what this condition is. But it fails to capture how distressing RLS can be. When you lie down to sleep or rest, you start feeling a maddening "creepy-crawly" sensation in your legs. Generally, the only way to stop it is to move the legs or walk around. Older people, pregnant women, and people with diabetes or lumbar disk disease are more susceptible. While causes are unknown, the high-risk groups all have low levels of magnesium. RLS symptoms are also associated with sugar, caffeine, and alcohol consumption, as well as some prescription drugs.

Run Out for Supplements

∼ Each day, take 500 milligrams of **magnesium**, 800 to 1,000 milligrams of **calcium**, and 800 to 1,000 milligrams of **potassium**. A shortage of any of these minerals can make your legs more twitchy.

∼ Drink mineral water that's high in **magnesium**. The optimum magnesium level is in the range of 100 milligrams per liter of water.

∼ Bump up your intake of **folic acid**, a B vitamin (also called folate). Folic acid helps build red blood cells, which in turn help oxygenate the body. That's an important benefit, since RLS is associated with a decrease in oxygen. Food sources of folic acid include leafy green vegetables, orange juice, and beans. You'll also find folate in most multivitamins.

∼ Eat **iron-rich** foods such as dark green vegetables, liver, wheat germ, kidney beans, and lean beef. Iron is part of the myoglobin molecule, which is a protein that stores oxygen in the muscles until it's needed. Without iron, myoglobin can't hold enough oxygen, and muscle problems may develop.

The Home Stretch

∼ When you get the urge to move your legs, start **rubbing** them, or **stretch** them to their full length and **point your toes**. These intentional movements send signals to your brain that can override the strange tingling sensations of RLS. But be sure to stop if the stretching produces a charley horse or leg cramps: Those are strong indications of magnesium deficiency and can't be alleviated by stretching.

⮑ Sit on the edge of the bed and firmly **massage** your calves to give the muscles deeper stimulation.

⮑ If those treatments don't calm your legs, get up and go for a brief **walk** around your home. Take long steps and bend your legs to stretch the muscles.

Before You Go to Bed

⮑ Sit in a tub filled with comfortably **hot water** for 10 to 15 minutes before you go to bed.

⮑ Chilling your legs may also help. Rub a **cold pack** on your legs before you go to bed.

⮑ Or combine the **heat and cold** treatments. Dip your legs in a comfortably hot bath for two minutes, then apply the cold pack to your legs for a minute. Repeat several times before bed.

Make Steady Progress

⮑ After you get into bed, practice the calming ritual known as **progressive muscle relaxation**. Breathe deeply for a few minutes, then tense the muscles in your feet. Hold the tension for a few seconds, then relax. Next, tense your calf muscles, hold, and relax. Then do the same with your thigh muscles. Repeat the tensing-and-relaxing pattern, working all the way up your body to your neck and face muscles. When you're finished, your whole body should feel relaxed.

Dip Into Homeopathy

⮑ Homeopathic doctors recommend **Causticum** at the 12C dilution for legs that are restless during the night.

⮑ Another option is a 12C dilution of **Tarentula hispanica**, three times a day until you see improvements in symptoms.

The Power of Prevention

⮑ In the evening, **avoid alcoholic or caffeinated drinks**, which stimulate the muscles and nerves in your legs.

⮑ Studies have found that **smokers** are more likely to have RLS than people who don't smoke.

⮑ **Avoid cold and sinus medications**, which can make RLS symptoms much worse.

Should I call **the doctor?**

If RLS is causing severe sleep loss or interfering with your work or daily activities, talk to your doctor. Because the condition is associated with mineral and vitamin deficiencies, you may also want to consult with a practitioner who specializes in nutrition, such as a naturopathic doctor.

Tried...

Drinking tonic water can quench those restless feelings in the legs.

...and true

This drink contains quinine, which does relieve symptoms in some people.

Ringworm

Any fungal infection spreads easily, and ringworm—once thought to be an actual worm lurking beneath the skin—is no exception. It all begins with prevention—keeping your feet and groin dry—and taking quick action with an over-the-counter antifungal medication when you see the first suggestion of an outbreak. Also try the home remedies below.

What's wrong

Ringworm is actually a fungal infection of the skin that tends to creep insidiously along the groin, scalp, feet, and face. It often starts out as a round, itchy red patch that grows outward. As it expands, the middle area heals, but all around is a red ring where infection continues to spread. If it's on your scalp, count on some flaky skin and patches of hair loss. The condition is contagious, thrives in warm, moist environments, and is often spread when people touch an infected surface such as a shower floor.

Use an Antifungal First

⮞ Look for over-the-counter **antifungal remedies** that contain ingredients such as miconazole, ketoconazole, clotrimazole, or terbinafine (Lamisil). Most need to be applied twice a day. If you follow the label directions, ringworm should start to clear within a week. Used twice a day for at least 8 weeks, OTCs like Zeasorb-AF powder—specifically for the feet and groin—are sure to get rid of the infection.

A Real Nut Case

⮞ If ringworm strikes in the fall, you might be able to resolve the problem with a green-hulled harvest from a nearby **black walnut** tree. Black walnuts have a distinctive-smelling thick green rind. Crush the rind into a pulp and apply it to ringworm up to four times a day until the condition clears up. (But that pulp is toxic if you eat it, so make sure it just goes on your skin.)

The Curry Cure

⮞ Turn ringworm away with **turmeric**. The main ingredient in curry powder, turmeric contains curcumin, which has helped many people who have inflammatory conditions like arthritis. It's not clear why turmeric should work so well on a fungal skin problem, but Asians have long used this spice to fight ringworm. Stir enough water into a teaspoon or two of powdered turmeric to make a paste. Smear it on the affected area and cover it with a bandage or piece of gauze. After 20 minutes to an hour, remove it. You can repeat this three or four times a day, but stop the treatment if turmeric irritates your skin.

Treat the Ring Right

- Be sure you keep the affected patch **clean and dry**.
- If the infection starts to ooze or blister over, apply cool or warm **moist compresses**. Or soak in water with dissolved **Epsom salt** or **Domeboro powder** to help dry the oozing rash. Take care not to break the blisters, and make an appointment with a doctor as soon as possible.

The Power of Prevention

- **Don't share shoes or used towels** with other people—they can spread an infection.
- If family members have ringworm, make sure that **no one shares clothing** or grooming items, such as **hairbrushes**.
- Wash in hot water any clothes, towels, washcloths, and bedclothes that may have come in touch with the infected area.
- Be sure to dry your feet completely soon after swimming or bathing, using a **hair dryer** whenever possible. The area between the toes is the most common place for fungus to start growing.
- Instead of going barefoot at a public swimming pool, wear **flip-flops** or **sandals** to avoid picking up fungus.
- Use a powder such as **Zeasorb-AF** in your shoes or your groin area to absorb excess moisture. The powder contains an antifungal ingredient for extra protection.
- Pets can carry ringworm that can be transferred to humans. If you see a **hairless spot on your dog or cat**, take your pet to the vet as soon as possible for a ringworm treatment.

Should I call **the doctor?**

If your symptoms don't improve after a few weeks of self-care treatments, or the ringworm continues to spread, talk to your doctor. If you have ringworm in the groin area, the doctor might prescribe an antifungal powder such as Nystatin. For ringworm of the scalp, you'll need to get a prescription drug that's taken orally. And if you have diabetes, it's essential to get ringworm treated by a doctor as soon as possible. It can cause skin cracking, and if bacteria enter the skin, you could end up with a serious infection.

Tick Off This Possibility

The ring created by the ringworm fungus resembles the "target" around a tick bite that's symptomatic of Lyme disease. So how can you tell the difference? If you're concerned, examine the "ring" area for some telltale signs. When ringworm has not yet been treated, it tends to be scaly, and the ring in the center is clear. Lyme disease, in its earliest stage, looks like a bull's-eye or target, and it has no scale. Also, if you have Lyme disease, the center of the ring is likely to be red or purplish at the site of the original tick bite.

Rosacea

You look like you're blushing, even when you're not. Or worse, you look like a teenager with a bad case of acne. Take heart. If Princess Diana could cope with her rosacea—you probably didn't even know she had it—so can you. Try these approaches to prevent mild flare-ups and flushing. Should your condition get worse, combine forces with a dermatologist to keep your ruddiness under control.

What's wrong

Sometimes rosacea looks no worse than a bothersome blush. But the condition can gradually worsen until it resembles severe acne. If you have rosacea, tiny blood vessels in the face widen and fill with blood until portions of the face seem suffused with red. The redness fades after a few hours, but if rosacea isn't treated, the face can take on a bumpy, sunburned look; blood vessels can become visible through the skin; and the nose may become red and enlarged.

A Wetting List

When your face gets warm and red, your first instinct is the right one: Cool it down. The easiest way is to soak a washcloth in **ice-cold water** and lay it on the red areas for about ten minutes. The cold tightens blood vessels.

Chamomile, applied to the skin, has anti-inflammatory effects. Rather than using chamomile oil, which is highly concentrated and might cause a skin reaction, use dilute tea. Steep several **chamomile tea** bags in three cups of boiling water for 10 minutes. Strain the liquid and chill it in the refrigerator. When your face is flushed, dip a cloth into the tea and apply it to the red area.

Wash on the Mild Side

Use a cleanser designed to be particularly gentle, such as **Cetaphil** or **Aquanil**, or **Dove soap for sensitive skin,** whenever you wash your face. You want to avoid soap that might be rough or irritating. What all these cleansers have in common is that they are moisturizing and contain no perfumes and few preservatives, which are the ingredients most likely to irritate skin.

Avoid any **exfoliating skin washes** or **acne cleansers**. These contain harsh ingredients, and acne treatments can actually make rosacea worse.

If you pick up a cleanser that lists **salicylic acid, benzoyl peroxide,** or **alcohol** as an ingredient, return it to the shelf—it will just **make rosacea worse**. Also steer clear of any abrasive cleaning products.

Avoid Face Flushers

⚘ **Give up** the spiciest of spicy foods, including such south-of-the-border treats as **hot sauce, chili, and jalapeño peppers**. After you eat such foods, your face not only feels like it's flushing, it is. The fine arteries expand in reaction to the spicy food.

⚘ **Alcohol also makes your blood vessels widen.** Take note of any flushing after you drink. If your face tends to turn redder when you've had a cocktail or a glass of beer or wine, opt for soda or water at the next social occasion.

⚘ **Stay out of hot tubs and saunas.** Their heat can trigger flushing of the skin on your face.

A Whiter Shade of Pale

⚘ Stay out of the direct sunlight as much as possible, particularly in the middle of the day when the sun is at its hottest. **Sunlight can lead to flare-ups of rosacea**, since it warms your skin, dilating the blood vessels in your face.

⚘ If you do have to be outside on a sunny day, wear a **wide-brimmed hat** that provides shade for your ears and cheeks as well as your nose. A baseball cap isn't enough.

⚘ Use **sunscreen**, and plenty of it. For anyone with rosacea, the best sunscreens contain **titanium dioxide** or **zinc oxide,** which physically block the sun's rays rather than absorbing them chemically.

Don't See Red

⚘ When tempers flare, so do blood vessels, and that can lead to an outbreak of rosacea. One of the best ways to keep a fiery response in check is simply to **count to ten**. Take it a step further by inhaling deeply as you count. Exhale fully while you count to ten again. After you've done this a few times, you'll find that you can handle the situation much more calmly.

Shaving Face

⚘ Men with rosacea need to take special care not to irritate their faces while attacking their whiskers. Use an **electric shaver** instead of razor blades. The shaver is less irritating.

⚘ If you use an aftershave, **stay away from** products that contain **alcohol, witch hazel**, or **menthol**.

Should I call **the doctor?**

Check with your doctor if you have the persistent skin reddening that is a sign of rosacea. Early diagnosis and treatment with prescription medicines (metronidazole-containing creams, sulfur-based face washes and creams, and oral antibiotics) can help prevent the condition from getting worse. So you'll want to see your doctor for treatment at the same time you take steps to stop outbreaks. For severe cases, a doctor might recommend a cauterization process involving electrical charges, or laser surgery.

Shingles

First step: Call your doctor, who will likely put you on a prescription antiviral drug. Meanwhile, you'll want all the relief you can get from the burning and pain. You can try acetaminophen or ibuprofen, plus the remedies in this chapter. But if the pain is more than you can stand, don't hesitate to call your doctor, who can prescribe stronger medication.

What's wrong

Shingles occurs when the dormant herpes zoster virus, which causes chicken pox, re-awakens in nerve cells and makes its way to the skin. About 20 percent of people who had chicken pox will later develop shingles, usually when they're over age 50. The infection causes a burning, blistering rash— often on the torso, face, and neck—which appears as a band or patch of raised dots. Itching, tingling, or pain can be mild or severe. Within a week or so, small, fluid-filled blisters form, dry up, and crust over. Anything that lowers resistance to infection, such as illness or stress, can awaken the virus. On average, the rash and pain last 2 to 4 weeks, but sometimes the pain lingers for months.

Beat the Blisters and Ditch the Itch

To help dry the blisters, apply **calamine lotion**. As the wet solution evaporates from your skin, it also draws moisture from the blisters.

If you have an **aloe vera** plant in your home or garden, cut a leaf and smooth the liquid over your skin. The milky liquid inside the leaves may help soothe the blisters. Or use an over-the-counter aloe vera gel (make sure it's 100% aloe).

A paste of **baking powder** and water will dry up blisters and soothe the itching. Add enough water to dry baking powder to create a paste, then apply it liberally to the affected area.

Another remedy for drying blisters and soothing inflammation is a paste made from **Epsom salt** and water. Apply directly to the affected area. Repeat as often as you wish.

Brew a tea of **lemon balm**, an herb from the mint family that European studies suggest fights herpes viruses. To make it, boil 2 teaspoons dried herb in 1 cup boiling water. Use a cotton ball to dab it directly onto the affected areas. Some herbalists recommend bolstering the brew with **rose oil** or mints such as **peppermint, spearmint**, and **sage**.

Reach into your pantry, where you probably have the ingredients for another shingles solution: **vinegar** and **honey**. Mix them together to form a paste and dab it onto your sores.

Send the Pain Packing

Dip a washcloth or towel into **cold water**, squeeze it out, and lay it over the affected area. Alternatively, you can use cold milk instead of water. Some people say that the milk is especially soothing.

⤳ Made from the extract of hot pepper, **capsaicin cream** can quell pain that lingers after the rash is gone. Zostrix is one brand to try. When you first put it on, you'll feel a burning sensation, but as long as you're not using it on an open rash, the burning will diminish as you continue using it over the next few weeks. (Just don't use the cream if the skin is broken or you have an open rash—it will burn intensely.)

⤳ If you still have pain after the blisters have healed, fill a bag with **ice** and use it to gently stroke your skin. Experts don't know why the cold treatment is helpful, but it does work.

Put Brakes on Breakouts

⤳ As long as you have your doctor's approval, take 500 to 1,000 milligrams of supplemental **lysine** three times a day during an outbreak. This amino acid prevents viruses from replicating and may speed healing.

⤳ Take two 250-milligram capsules of **echinacea** three times a day to help your body fight the infection.

⤳ Try taking **cat's claw**, an herb long used for a variety of purposes among indigenous people of Peru and now considered a promising treatment for viral disorders, including shingles. Follow the dosage directions on the package.

The Power of Prevention

⤳ To protect others from the virus, **wash your hands often**, especially if you have an oozing rash. The blisters contain the varicella virus, so you could infect someone with chicken pox. Or cover the blisters with an antibiotic ointment and wrap them with gauze.

Should I call **the doctor?**

Yes, and quickly. You should contact the doctor within 72 hours if you develop the typical symptoms. Starting antiviral drugs immediately can help reduce the severity and duration of an attack and may also stave off postherpetic neuralgia, the painful aftereffects of shingles. Call, too, if you're unable to endure the pain of a current outbreak of shingles, or if your shingles have disappeared but the pain hasn't. If you get shingles on your nose, forehead, or anywhere else near your eyes, call your doctor immediately for treatment, as there is a risk of going blind.

Pain After the Pain

Many people who develop shingles experience lingering pain in the affected area months or even years after an attack. This is called postherpetic neuralgia (PHN). If you have PHN, be sure to see your doctor, who can prescribe a medication such as Neurontin (gabapentin), an effective oral drug approved for shingles. Other possible treatments include the Lidoderm patch, which feeds medication into damaged nerves under the skin, and an injection with local anesthetic to block pain signals.

Sinusitis

You're stuffed up, your face hurts, and the pressure is getting to you. If a bacterial infection is the cause of your sinusitis, your doctor can give you antibiotics that will help. Otherwise, oral or nasal decongestants can give you temporary relief. (Don't use them for more than three days or the swelling in your sinuses could get worse.) Of course, you don't have to dash off to the drugstore every time your sinuses swell. There are plenty of other ways to reopen blocked passages and help yourself feel better.

What's **wrong**

The sinuses—air-filled cavities on either side of the nose—are lined with a superthin mucous membrane. When the membrane becomes inflamed and infected, it swells, blocking channels that allow mucus to drain into the nose. The resulting pressure can cause headache, nasal congestion, yellow-green nasal discharge, and cheekbone pain. Sinusitis that lasts three weeks or less (acute sinusitis) may result from a bacterial infection, a cold or the flu, or swimming in contaminated water. Chronic sinusitis is often caused by a deviated septum, irritation from dust or cigarette smoke, or fungal infections.

Do Some Steam Cleaning

⚬ **Steam** can relieve the painful sinus pressure. Take a long, hot shower, inhale the steam, and let the water spray on your face. Then snort and swallow the hot water until your sinuses are clear.

⚬ Give your congested sinuses a mentholated steam treatment. Boil a pot of water to which you've added a few drops of **eucalyptus oil**, then remove the pot from the stove. Drape a towel over your head and shoulders, then lean forward so it forms a tent over the pan. Keep your face about 18 inches above the water as you breathe in deeply. As the vapor rises, it carries droplets of oil into your sinuses and loosens secretions.

⚬ Don't have any eucalyptus oil on hand? No problem. Just add a teaspoon of **Vicks VapoRub** to the water instead.

Sniff a Salt Solution

⚬ Another method of loosening mucus and reducing swelling is irrigating the sinuses with a **saline solution**. Make the salt solution by mixing one-third teaspoon of table salt and a pinch of baking soda in a cup of warm water. Then fill an ear-bulb syringe with the solution. Closing one nostril with your thumb, tilt your head back and squirt the solution into one nostril while you sniff. Blow your nose gently, then repeat with the other nostril.

⚬ You can also use a device called a **neti pot**, available at health-food stores. (It looks like a small watering can with a narrow spout.). To use the neti pot, place half the liquid in the device. Standing over a sink, place the spout into one nostril, then tilt your head to the side and down, away from the spout. Pour the saline solution into the nostril. The liquid will come out of the other nostril. Once it has drained out, blow your nose gently into a tissue. Repeat with the other nostril using the other half of the saline solution.

Heat Those Cavities

⌒ Inhale freshly grated **horseradish**. The pungent root contains a fiery substance that helps to thin mucus.

⌒ Alternatively, mix equal amounts of grated **horseradish** and **lemon juice** and eat 1 teaspoonful an hour before breakfast. Take another teaspoonful an hour before dinner.

⌒ If you're a fan of spicy-hot foods, add some chili peppers to your meals. The peppers contain **capsaicin**, a compound that breaks up congestion and promotes the drainage of mucus. And when you're all out of chilis, you can sprinkle on cayenne pepper instead; it, too, has all-powerful capsaicin.

⌒ Many studies show that a substance in **garlic** called allicin is a potent antibacterial and natural antibiotic. Crush 1 clove of garlic, drop it into a quarter-cup of water, and swish it around. Then use an eyedropper to extract some of this garlic water and put 10 drops in each nostril. At the end of 3 days, your infection should be well on its way to healing.

Enter the Land of Ahhhs

⌒ A cup of hot **tea** can help thin nasal mucus. **Chamomile tea** was once considered a folk remedy for sinusitis. If you like it, try it. Another herbal tea to try is Red Zinger from Celestial Seasonings. We heard that one opera singer swears by it for sinus problems. It contains rosehips and lemongrass. Drink several cups a day as soon as you feel an infection coming on.

⌒ **Get plenty of rest**. When you're lying down, however, be sure to keep a pillow under your head to help your sinuses drain. Lying flat on your back without a pillow can make your congestion worse.

⌒ Apply a **warm washcloth** over your eyes and cheekbones. Leave it in place until the cloth cools. Then warm it up again and repeat as often as needed until you get some relief.

Should I call **the doctor?**

Usually sinusitis responds well to self-treatment. But in rare cases the condition can turn serious. Call your doctor immediately if you feel pain or have paralysis in your eyes, or if they bulge or turn red. Also tell your doctor if you have nausea and vomiting. In very rare cases, the infection may spread to the eyes or the brain, possibly leading to vision loss, meningitis, or brain abscess.

Become a Nose Masseur

Giving your sinuses a **mini-massage** will increase blood circulation to the area and help to chase away the pain. Using your index fingers, press hard on the outer edge of your nostrils at the base of the nose.

Another pressure-relieving move: Apply your thumbs to both sides of your nose, about halfway up, and press firmly on the cartilage. Hold for 30 seconds, then release. You can repeat this as often as you like.

For sinus relief using **acupressure**, use your left thumb and index finger to press the areas next to the inner eyes on both sides of the bridge of your nose. At the same time, use your fingers and the heel of your other hand to grab muscles on both sides of the spine at the back of your neck. Put pressure on all four points for about one minute.

Bring In the Herbal Bouncers

Echinacea and **astragalus** are two herbs that can boost immunity and sometimes banish bacteria and viruses. For echinacea the recommended dosage is 200 milligrams standardized to 3.5% echinacosides, taken four times a day. Astragalus capsules should also be 200 milligrams, standardized to 0.5% glucosides and 70% polysaccharides. Take astragalus twice a day between meals. If you have the kind of sinusitis that comes on suddenly after a cold or flu, take the full dosage of both these herbs for a few weeks or until the sinusitis gets better. For chronic sinusitis—the kind that drags on and on—alternate taking echinacea one week and astragalus the next.

Try taking 250 to 500 milligrams of **goldenseal** three times a day. This herb is thought to fight infections and is

New Flight Plan

Some frequent fliers have problems on the way up; others, on the way down. When a plane takes off, air pressure is reduced and the pressure builds in your head, blocking your sinuses (or the Eustachian tubes in your ears). In mid-flight you might be all right, but on the way down, the pressure changes again, and your sinuses take the punishment. To avoid the pain, use a decongestant nasal spray or ask your doctor about a prescription inhaler you can use before you endure the ups and downs of another flight.

sometimes combined with echinacea. Goldenseal tea can be either drunk or used as a nasal wash. To make it, boil one-half to one gram of goldenseal in a cup of water. Don't use goldenseal for more than one or two weeks at a time, though.

The Power of Prevention

⬧ Run a **cold-mist humidifier** in your bedroom at night to keep your nasal and sinus passages from drying out. Just make sure you clean the humidifier once a week so mildew or fungi can't set up shop.

⬧ **Cut down on** your consumption of **alcoholic beverages**. Alcohol causes swelling of nasal and sinus membranes.

⬧ **Avoid swimming in a chlorinated pool**—and never dive. Chlorine irritates the lining of the nose and sinuses. Diving forces water from nasal passages up into the sinuses.

⬧ **Stay away from smoke-filled rooms**. Cigarette smoke dries out nasal passages, and bacteria get trapped in the sinuses.

Snoring

If you're the snorer in your household, lucky you. After all, you're the only one who can sleep right through the thunderous racket. For the sake of household harmony, show your partner the tips in the "Self-Defense" sidebar (page 218). Then try the following preventive measures. Changing your sleeping position may be all it takes, but a larger project—namely, losing weight—is often the real ticket to tranquil nights.

What's **wrong**

When you snore, structures in the mouth and throat—the tongue, upper throat, soft palate, and uvula—vibrate against the tonsils and adenoids. There are many possible causes. Overweight people are more likely to snore, and experts think it's because the extra fatty tissue compresses the air passages. Drinking alcohol before bedtime is another factor: It causes throat muscles to relax and tissues to sag. And whenever you have nasal congestion from a cold or allergies, you're more likely to snore because inflamed tissues and extra mucus interfere with airflow.

Put Yourself in a Good Position

➤ Buy yourself a few extra pillows and **prop yourself up** in bed, rather than lying flat on your back. You'll prevent the tissues in your throat from falling into your air passages.

➤ **Elevate** the head of your bed. An easy way to do it is to place several flat boards under the legs at the top end of the bed. A couple of short lengths of two-by-eights or two-by-tens under each leg should raise the bed enough to do the trick.

➤ **Sleep on your side**. Of course, there's no guarantee you'll stay in that position, but at least start on your side with your arms wrapped around a pillow. There's a good reason you don't want to sleep on your back: In that position, your tongue and soft palate rest against the back of your throat, blocking the airway.

➤ If hugging a pillow doesn't help, you can ace the problem with service from a sewn-in **tennis ball**. Here's how: Sew a little pouch on the back of your pajama top and tuck a tennis ball inside. At night, if you start to roll on your back while you're sleeping, you'll get a nudge from that tennis ball, prompting you to get back on your side.

Don't Be So Nosy

➤ If nasal congestion is causing your snoring, take a **decongestant** or **antihistamine** before you turn in.

➤ Tape your nose open with **nasal strips**, available at most drugstores. They may look odd, but who's watching? Following the directions on the package, tape one of the strips to the outside of your nose before you fall asleep. They'll lift and open your nostrils to increase airflow.

 Gargle with a **peppermint mouthwash** to shrink the lining of your nose and throat. This is especially effective if your snoring is a temporary condition caused by a head cold or an allergy. To mix up the herbal gargle, add one drop of peppermint oil to a glass of cold water. (But *only* gargle—do not swallow.)

Chin Up

 It sounds extreme, but some people have used a **neck brace**—the kind people with whiplash wear—to stop their snoring. It works by keeping your chin extended so your throat doesn't bend and your airway stays open. You don't have to use a stiff plastic brace, however. A soft foam one, available at drugstores or medical supply stores, is less restraining and will work just as well.

Axe Allergies

 Reduce bedroom allergens (dust, pet dander, mold) to alleviate nasal stuffiness by **vacuuming floors and drapes**. Change sheets and pillowcases often.

 If your snoring is a seasonal problem—and you know you're allergic to pollen—try drinking up to three cups of tea made from the herb **stinging nettle**. Herbalists recommend it for soothing inflammation caused by pollen allergies. To make the tea, pour 1 cup boiling water over 1 tablespoon of the dried leaf (available in health-food stores). Cover the tea and let it steep for 5 minutes. Strain and drink. Drink one cup of tea just before bedtime.

Watch Your Mouth

 Don't eat a heavy meal or drink alcoholic beverages within three hours of turning in. Both can cause your throat muscles to relax more than normal.

 Snoring improves as you **shed some weight**. Losing 10 percent of your body weight can help by easing constriction of the upper airway.

Should I call **the doctor?**

Loud, excessive snoring can signal sleep apnea, a potentially dangerous condition that requires treatment. Contact your doctor if you're a loud snorer who stops breathing for short periods when you're asleep. You should also notify the doctor if you sometimes wake up gasping for breath, if you wake up with headaches, or if you're sleepy during the day. Sleep apnea can reduce levels of oxygen in the blood, eventually leading to elevated blood pressure and an enlarged heart. In addition to lifestyle modifications (losing weight or changing your sleeping position), some doctors sometimes recommend a continuous positive airway pressure (CPAP) device for nightly use. Surgery is also possible.

A Short Course in Snoring Self-Defense

If you're living with someone who snores, there's a better than even chance the nightly sonorities are fraying your relationship. But remember, other spouses and partners have dealt with this too—and survived. So before you head for the hills, consider some practical methods to deal with the rumblings of your otherwise lovable bedmate.

- Buy yourself a pair of earplugs. They are inexpensive and quite comfortable, once you get accustomed to them.
- A white-noise machine can make nights with a snorer more bearable. These electronic devices produce a consistent sound that muffles other noises.
- Turn in well before your snoring spouse. That way, at least, you have a head start on a good night's sleep. Some well-practiced partners can sleep right through the full-scale thunder of Rip Van Winkle.

Quit smoking. Tobacco smoke irritates mucous membranes, so your throat swells, narrowing the airway. Smokers also have more problems with nasal congestion.

If you're regularly taking any kind of **medication**, talk to your doctor about alternatives. Some drugs can make snoring worse, including sleeping pills and sedatives.

Dry air can contribute to snoring. There are lots of ways to do battle with dry air. A **humidifier** or **steam vaporizer** in the bedroom can keep your air passages moist; just be sure to clean it regularly, following the manufacturer's instructions. Another approach: Just before bedtime, fill a bowl with hot water, drape a towel over your head, bend over the bowl so your nose is roughly six inches from the water, and breathe deeply through your nose for a few minutes.

Sties

Perhaps the biggest challenge when you have a sty in your eye is resisting the temptation to rub it. It's a natural reaction, but no amount of rubbing will get rid of that something-in-my-eye feeling, and the bacteria that infected the follicle can spread to others. Instead, use moist heat to bring the sty to a head. And follow our tips to keep your eyelids clean and clear of future irritations.

Have a Heated Exchange

⤳ Apply a **warm compress** to the affected eye for 10 to 15 minutes four times a day for two or three days. For a compress, you can use a soft washcloth, a piece of clean cotton cloth, a gauze pad, or even a tea bag. Run warm water over the item, close your eye, and hold the moistened compress against the eyelid. Once you get used to the heat against your eye, you can moisten the compress a few more times with ever-warmer water. The heat will cause a sty to come to a head and rupture sooner. Once you've used a compress, it should either be thrown away or (if it's a washcloth) washed in very hot water before you use it again. Otherwise, you might re-infect your eye with the bacteria.

⤳ To give a hot compress extra infection-fighting power, soak it in tea made from **calendula** flowers. Put 2 teaspoons dried flowers in a bowl, add 2 cups boiling water, and steep for 20 minutes. Then strain out the flowers.

⤳ There's another way to bring heat to a painful peeper. Boil an **egg** until it's hardboiled, then take it out of the hot water and wrap it in a clean cloth. Hold the hot egg against the outside of your eyelid. It stays hot longer than the compress. (And when you're done, you can make an egg salad sandwich out of your sty remedy.)

⤳ Hot **potatoes** work too (but not as leftovers). Microwave a potato, cut it in half, and put it on a cloth over your eye. It stays hot for a long time, so you can relax, recline, and enjoy the break.

What's **wrong**

Sties are red, inflamed, painful bumps on the upper or lower edge of the eyelid that look much like pimples. They occur when an eyelash follicle gets clogged with dirt or oil, then infected by bacteria. (If a gland on the eyelid is clogged, you have a chalazion instead of a sty.) Your eye may water, or you may feel like there's something in it. Normally, a sty enlarges with pus over the course of several days, then ruptures and heals. The sty may disappear completely once the infection is over, or it may leave a small fluid-filled cyst that requires medical treatment.

When Is a Sty Not a Sty?

A chalazion—an enlarged, blocked oil gland in the eyelid—looks like a sty for the first few days, but it becomes larger and lasts longer. You can tell it's not a sty because it's farther from the edge of the eyelid, and it's likely to turn into a hard, painless, round bump. Most chalazions go away with lots of hot compresses that melt the thickened oil and allow it to drain from the pores of the eyelid. But if it lingers for weeks or months, you might want to visit your doctor for a steroid cream or antibiotics that will help it heal. In some cases, doctors recommend minor surgery to remove chalazions.

Should I call the doctor?

Although sties are painful and annoying, they're usually harmless. Call a doctor if the sty starts to bleed, grows very large very quickly, or doesn't begin to heal after two days. You may have a more serious eyelid infection called cellulitis.

Beat Back Bacteria

➤ To boost your immune system and help fight infection-causing bacteria, take 200 milligrams of **echinacea** three or four times a day and continue until the sty goes away.

➤ Eat one clove of fresh **garlic** a day. It may not be your favorite appetizer, but it has antibacterial properties. If you can stand to, eat it raw for best effect.

The Power of Prevention

➤ If you are prone to sties, you may want to bathe your eyelids once a day to keep the follicles clear. An easy way to do this is to gently rinse your closed eyelids with a mixture of **no-tears baby shampoo** and warm water.

➤ Every couple of days, apply a **warm compress** to your eyelids to prevent oil glands from becoming blocked.

➤ Take a tablespoon of **flaxseed oil** every day, or take two flaxseed-oil capsules. It can help prevent follicles from clogging. If you want to get the most benefit from pure flaxseed oil, add it to salads or put it on bread, but don't cook it. Heat breaks down its nutrients.

➤ To prevent spreading infection to other members of your family—or re-infecting yourself—when you have a sty, **wash your hands frequently** and keep them away from your eyes. For the same reason, **don't share your washcloths** or towels with other family members. Change your towel and pillowcase often.

➤ Make sure you get enough **vitamin A** by taking a multivitamin or eating foods such as broccoli, cantaloupe, spinach, and swordfish. If sties are a problem for you, it may be a sign of vitamin A deficiency.

Sunburn

If you have the complexion of boiled lobster and you're in significant pain, take aspirin, ibuprofen, or some other over-the-counter anti-inflammatory drug to reduce the swelling and relieve the pain. And of course, do what you'd do for any other type of burn: Cool it with cold water to stop the sizzle. You may also want to use one of the sunburn sprays, sold in the drugstore, that contain numbing ingredients. Finally, make sure to learn your lesson and remember to wear sunscreen next time you venture out into the sun.

Dip In

For immediate relief, soak the sunburned areas in **cold water** (but not ice water) or with cold compresses for 15 minutes. The cold reduces swelling and wicks away heat from your skin.

If you're burned all over, take a soak in a cool bath to which you've added **oatmeal**. You can either buy a colloidal oatmeal product such as Aveeno or simply grind up a cup of oatmeal in a food processor and add it to your bath.

Brew up a pot of **green tea** and let it cool. Soak a clean cloth in the tea, and use it as a compress. The tea contains ingredients that help protect the skin from ultraviolet radiation damage and reduce inflammation.

Use the cooling, aromatic qualities of **peppermint** to quell the scorch of a sunburn. Either make peppermint tea or mix two drops of peppermint oil with a cup of lukewarm water. Chill the concoction and gently bathe the burned area.

Pantry Painkillers

For extra-painful spots of sunburn, rub the area gently with sliced **cucumber** or **potato**. They contain compounds that cool the burn and help reduce swelling.

Vinegar contains acetic acid—one of the components of aspirin. It can help ease sunburn pain, itching, and inflammation. Soak a few sheets of paper towels in white vinegar, and

What's wrong

The outer layers of your skin have become inflamed by overexposure to the sun's ultraviolet (UV) rays. With a first-degree burn, the skin may be hot and tender as well. Small, fluid-filled blisters indicate second-degree sunburn. Worst of all are third-degree burns, which cause blistering, red or purple skin discoloration, chills, fever, nausea, and headache. With repeated severe sunburns, your skin ages more rapidly, and risk of skin cancer increases. Fair-haired people with light skin are more at risk for sunburn, as are those who take certain medications such as sulfa drugs, some antibiotics, and oral diabetes medications.

Should I call
the doctor?

Most sunburns are first-degree burns. The pain will ease in one to four days. But call the doctor if your sunburned skin starts to blister, you run a fever or develop chills or nausea, or if the pain becomes unbearable.

Tried...

Many people report that putting milk on a sunburn is extremely soothing.

...and true

Milk has a high fat content, and it doesn't seal the skin the way lard does. If your burn feels cooler that way, go ahead and milk the remedy for all it's worth.

apply them to the burned areas. Leave them on until the towels are dry. Repeat as needed.

⟡ If the sunburn itches, take a cool bath, but add 2 cups of **vinegar** to the bathwater before you get in.

Put On a Coating

⟡ Mix **baking soda** and **vinegar** to make a thick paste, and slather it over the sunburned areas. Apply the salve before bedtime, and leave it on overnight.

⟡ Sprinkle your sheets with **cornstarch** to minimize painful chafing. (Use this technique only for bad sunburns, since you'll have to wash the sheets afterward.)

⟡ Apply a light coating of pure **aloe vera** to the painful skin, using either a fresh piece from the plant or in the gel form you can buy at the drugstore. If you buy the gel, make sure it's 100% pure aloe vera.

⟡ Try applying an oil or ointment of **St. John's wort** as a burn balm: The herb has antiseptic and painkilling properties, and is thought to help heal skin wounds. If you're taking the herb internally, however, stay out of the sun: It makes skin more sensitive to damaging rays.

The Power of Prevention

⟡ Always slather your skin with a **sunscreen** that contains a sun protection factor (SPF) of 15 or higher, at least 30 minutes before going outdoors. Insist that your loved ones do the same.

⟡ Between 10 A.M. and 3 P.M., **limit your exposure to the sun**. This is when the sun's rays are at their strongest.

⟡ If you burn easily or have been diagnosed with skin cancer in the past, take no chances: **Cover up in the sun**. That means long pants, long sleeves, a wide-brimmed hat, and sunglasses.

Swimmer's Ear

"But I'm not a swimmer!" you say. You don't have to be. The infection can get started when you're just taking a shower. But you can be quite sure it's swimmer's ear if you feel a piercing pain when you push on the triangular flap that covers the opening to the ear canal. To deal with the pain, your easiest option is an over-the-counter painkiller such as aspirin or acetaminophen. Also try heat to ease the ache and take steps (described below) to dry out the ear canal and make it unfriendly to the bacteria or fungi that caused the infection.

Warming the Cockles

～ For soothing relief, treat your ear to heat. Use a **hot-water bottle** or a **heating pad** set on low. If you're using the bottle, wrap it in a towel so it feels comfortably warm, not super hot. If you're using a heating pad, for safety's sake, be careful not to fall asleep with that electric pad nestled against your ear.

Drop In Center

～ Take advantage of garlic's potent antibacterial properties and use this herb in eardrops. You can buy **garlic oil** in health-food stores, or make your own. Grate three medium cloves of garlic and place them in a shallow dish. Cover them with olive oil and let the mixture stand overnight. Strain out the garlic and apply 3 drops in the affected ear.

～ If your infection itches but doesn't hurt, mix equal parts of **rubbing alcohol** with **distilled white vinegar**, and use a clean eyedropper to put a few drops in your ear. Tilt your head so the mixture flows into the ear canal, then tug your earlobe to make sure it flows all the way in. Keep your head tilted (or lie down) for a few minutes, then sit erect and tilt your ear toward your shoulder to let the excess drain out. (You'll need a tissue or handkerchief to catch the runoff.) Because vinegar creates an acid environment—inhospitable to bacteria and fungi—it helps to clear infection. And the drops also help dry

What's **wrong**

Swimmer's ear is an infection of the outer ear canal. It happens when water gets trapped in your ears and allows bacteria or fungi to flourish. At first, the affected ear feels blocked and may itch. If you leave it untreated, the infection can cause swelling, accompanied by some drainage of fluid. The condition can be quite painful. Often, the area that hurts the most is the triangular piece of cartilage called the tragus that covers the front of the ear canal.

Usually swimmer's ear is easy to treat and goes away, never to be heard from again. But not always. In about one percent of all cases, it comes back again no matter what you do to prevent a recurrence. Some particularly hard-to-treat bacteria has set up home in your ear, and all you can do is try to keep it under control. If you have this problem, be sure to keep your doctor informed. In rare cases, the infection can spread into nearby tissue around the ear (a severe condition called malignant otitis externa). People with diabetes and those with compromised immune systems are most susceptible.

Should I call **the doctor?**

If you've ever had a ruptured eardrum or had tubes put in your ears, see your doctor for any kind of earache. Otherwise, you can usually treat a mild case of swimmer's ear at home. But if you develop sudden, severe ear pain, or hearing loss, get to the doctor. You'll also need a doctor's help if you have signs or symptoms of a punctured eardrum (blood, discharge from the ear, very intense pain followed by sudden relief). For swimmer's ear that doesn't respond to home remedies, a doctor can prescribe antibiotics.

out the ear canal, because they contain alcohol, which evaporates rapidly.

꙾ If your ear is painful, skip the alcohol. Just use **vinegar** blended with a few drops of water.

꙾ If your ear itches, mix a few drops of **lavender oil** with a teaspoon of **olive oil** and rub the mixture in your outer ear. You don't need to use much.

The Power of Prevention

꙾ Wear wax or silicone **earplugs**, available at most drugstores, to keep your ears dry when you're swimming or showering. The earplugs can be softened and shaped to fit snugly into your outer ear canal.

꙾ After you swim or shower, shake your head to remove any water that remains in your ears. Better yet, gently **blow-dry** your ears. Pull the flap of your ear to create an open airway to your ear canal. Set the hair dryer on the lowest setting and direct the airstream into your ear for 30 seconds. The nozzle of the hair dryer should be about 18 inches away.

꙾ Dilute a small amount of **apple cider vinegar** with an equal amount of **distilled water** and use 1 drop in each ear after you swim or shower. The vinegar is good for preventing bacterial and fungal infections as well as clearing them up.

꙾ Don't try to get all the wax out of your ears. In normal amounts, earwax coats the ear canal, which protects your inner ear from moisture.

Teeth Grinding

You had a stressful day and you unleashed your tension by grinding your teeth at night—maybe grinding so forcefully that you woke up the household. And perhaps you paid the price the next day with a headache. For head and facial pain caused by teeth grinding (also called bruxism), you can get temporary relief from over-the-counter pain relievers like aspirin or acetaminophen. But that doesn't get to the root of the problem. For that you'll want to consult with your dentist. In the meantime, here are some ways to minimize the daily (or nightly) grind.

Enjoy Your Retiring

➤ **Avoid stressful thoughts, activities, and movies** in the hours before bedtime. You probably don't realize it, but just before bed is the worst time to pay the bills, watch *Die Hard* reruns, or talk about your in-laws. Get to your finances, violent movies, and sensitive subjects early in the evening. If you are bothered by worries, jot down things that you need to address the next day. Then take a **long, warm bath** before you go to bed.

➤ While you're in the bath—or even when you're lying in bed—cover your jaw with a washcloth that's been soaked in hot water. The extra warmth will relax your jaw muscles.

➤ Practice **progressive muscle relaxation** before you go to sleep, so tension doesn't lead you to grind at night. When you're lying in bed, tense, then relax the muscles in your feet. Repeat with your calf muscles, then thigh muscles, and so on, progressively tensing and relaxing each set of muscles all the way up your body. By the time you tense and relax your neck and jaw muscles, you should feel as limp as a rag doll.

➤ **Avoid eating within an hour of bedtime.** Digesting food while you sleep makes you more likely to grind your teeth.

Be Guarded

➤ A protective **mouth guard** made for boxers and defensive linebackers will work for teeth grinders too. Many types of protective mouth guards are available at sporting-goods

What's **wrong**

You may respond to stressful situations during the day by clenching or grinding your teeth at night, without even realizing you're doing it. This presents a problem, since your teeth are designed to touch briefly when you're chewing and swallowing. They aren't built for the punishment of constant grinding. Common triggers are tension and anger. Nighttime grinding can lead to cracked teeth and headaches, as well as the neck and jaw pain called temporomandibular disorder (TMD).

If you wake up with
pain in your jaw, neck,
or shoulder, or have
morning headaches,
talk to your dentist or
doctor. This is particularly
important if your
bedmate reports that you
grind your teeth at night.
And you need to see the
doctor immediately if you
have a broken tooth from
the grinding. For severe
teeth grinding, you can be
fitted with a very effective
appliance called the NTI-
tss (nociceptive trigeminal
inhibition–tension
suppression system). It
protects you from the
damaging and often
migraine-producing
clenching on back molars.

Did you
know?

When you grind, you may
be putting as much as
1,200 pounds of pressure
on the crowns and roots.
That recurring pressure is
what can break or loosen
your teeth.

stores. Follow directions on how to mold it to your bite, then wear it to bed at night. The rubbery material will absorb pressure and save your teeth from damage. (If you find that the mouth guard keeps falling out, or you wear it right through, talk to your dentist about a customized mouth guard.)

Give Your Jaw a Break

During the day, make a conscious point of **keeping your jaw relaxed and your teeth apart**. As a reminder to yourself, rest your tongue between your top and lower teeth—so if you start to bite down, you'll chomp on some nerve endings. Doctors have observed that people who can break the daytime teeth-grinding habit are less likely to do it unconsciously at night.

Avoid excessively hard or chewy foods—not only gum and hard candy, but also steak or dried foods that require a lot of jaw action. And if you're in the habit of chewing on the end of your pencil, try to stop. When you work your jaws during the day, the pattern is likely to continue in your sleep.

Watch What You Imbibe

Keep alcohol consumption to a minimum—or, better yet, stop drinking altogether. This is especially important in the evening. Though sleep experts aren't sure why, people who drink heavily at night are more likely to grind their teeth when they sleep.

Avoid caffeinated drinks. Since caffeine is a stimulant, if you drink coffee, black tea, or caffeinated soft drinks, you're far more likely to grind your teeth.

Get Mineral Power

Take powdered **calcium** and **magnesium**—in a two-to-one ratio—every day. These minerals help your jaw muscles relax, particularly at night. Dosages range from 600 milligrams of calcium along with 300 milligrams of magnesium to 1,000 milligrams of calcium with 500 milligrams of magnesium daily. Start at the lower dose, and if you don't get relief after a couple of weeks, increase the dosages. Calcium/magnesium tablets are also available, but they don't dissolve as readily. When you use the powdered form, dissolve the mineral supplements in an acidic liquid like orange or grapefruit juice.

Toothache

Toothaches range from throbbing to excruciating, but with a good dentist as your ally, the pain should be short-lived. If you can't get an appointment right away, you can stop at the pharmacy for a pain-relieving gel like Anbesol or Orajel. (The active ingredient they have in common is benzocaine—the same topical pain reliever is found in products that relieve sunburn.) For general pain relief, you can also take aspirin or acetaminophen (Tylenol). And try the following approaches.

Get Cloves to the Pain

⌇ Dab some **clove oil** directly on your bad tooth. Clove oil has remarkable bacteria-slaying properties—and it also has a numbing effect, which is why it's a longtime folk remedy for toothache. In the 1800s, when toothpaste was scant and dentists employed tools of torture, every doctor carried a good supply of clove oil. Today we know that this extract from the clove bud contains eugenol, which acts as a local anesthetic. The oil may sting at first, but then blissful relief sets in.

⌇ You can get the same numbing effect from **whole cloves**. Put a few in your mouth, let them moisten until they soften, bruise them a bit between your non-hurting molars to release their oil, then hold the softened cloves against your painful tooth for up to half an hour.

⌇ If you don't have any cloves, make a paste of **powdered ginger** and **red (cayenne) pepper**. Pour the powdered ingredients in the bottom of a cup, then add a drop or two of water to make the paste. Roll a small ball of cotton into enough paste to saturate it, and place it on your painful tooth. (This can irritate the gums, so keep the cotton on the tooth.) In addition to using the spices together, you can try them separately. Either one can help relieve tooth pain.

Swish Channels

⌇ Rinse your mouth with a **tincture of myrrh**. The astringent effects help with inflammation, and myrrh offers the

What's wrong

Cavities often cause tooth pain, and you get cavities from bacteria in the mouth that are thriving on sugary and starchy foods that cling to teeth and gums. The bacteria produce acids that damage your teeth, and when the damage reaches a nerve, misery sets in. But there can be other causes as well—a filling that's come loose, a cracked tooth, an abscess (a pocket of infection at the gum line), or a sinus condition. Any infection that reaches the root is sure to cause pain.

Should I call the doctor?

Whatever else you do, make an appointment to see your dentist. The home remedies in this chapter can provide temporary relief, but your dentist needs to do some exploration and find out what's causing this toothache. Odds are, you have a problem that requires treatment. If you don't find out what's causing the ache, it will only get worse.

added benefit of killing bacteria. Simmer 1 teaspoon of powdered myrrh in 2 cups water for 30 minutes. Strain and let cool. Rinse with 1 teaspoon of the solution in a half-cup water five to six times a day.

~ **Peppermint** tea has a nice flavor and some numbing power. Put 1 teaspoon dried peppermint leaves in 1 cup boiling water and steep for 20 minutes. After the tea cools, swish it around in your mouth, then spit it out or swallow. Repeat as often as needed.

~ To help kill bacteria and relieve some discomfort, swish with a mouthful of **3% hydrogen peroxide solution.** This can provide temporary relief if the toothache is accompanied by fever and a foul taste in the mouth (both are signs of infection), but like other toothache remedies, it's only a stopgap measure until you see your dentist and get the source of infection cleared up. A hydrogen peroxide solution is only for rinsing. Spit it out, then rinse several times with plain water.

~ Stir a teaspoon of **salt** into a glass of warm water and rinse for up to 30 seconds before you spit it out. Salt water cleanses the area around the tooth and draws out some of the fluid that causes swelling. Repeat this treatment as often as needed.

Compresses for Comfort

~ Place a small **ice cube** in a plastic bag, wrap a thin cloth around the bag, and apply it to the aching tooth for about 15 minutes to numb the nerves. Alternatively, that ice pack can go on your cheek, over the painful tooth.

~ A warm, wet **tea bag** is a standard folk remedy for toothache that's worth a try. Black tea contains astringent tannins, which may reduce swelling and give you temporary relief.

~ Another country cure calls for soaking a small piece of **brown paper** (from a grocery or lunch bag) in **vinegar,** sprinkling one side with **black pepper,** and holding this to the cheek. The warm sensation on your cheek may distract you from your tooth pain.

A Gentle Brush-Off

~ Use a **toothpaste that's designated "for sensitive teeth."** If you have a problem with shrinking gums, this could relieve a lot of the pain you probably experience from hot or cold foods. When gums shrink, the dentin beneath your teeth's enamel surface is exposed, and this material is particularly sensitive.

🔊 Switch to the **softest-bristled brush** you can find to help preserve gum tissue and prevent further shrinking.

Caulk It

🔊 If you've broken a tooth or have lost a filling, you can relieve some pain by covering the exposed area with softened **chewing gum**. This might work with a loose filling, too, to hold it in place until you can get to the dentist. To avoid further discomfort, avoid chewing anything with that tooth until you can have it repaired.

Press Here for Relief

🔊 Try an **acupressure** technique to stop tooth pain fast. With your thumb, press the point on the back of your other hand where the base of your thumb and your index finger meet. Apply pressure for about two minutes. This helps trigger the release of endorphins, the brain's feel-good hormones. (*Off-limits* . . . if you're pregnant.)

Tried...

According to folklore, if you massage your hand with an ice cube, you can help relieve a toothache.

...and true

When nerves in your fingers send "cold" signals to your brain, they may override the pain signals coming from your tooth. Just wrap up an ice cube in a thin cloth and massage it in the fleshy area between your thumb and forefinger.

Ulcers

This is one of those ailments that make us all too happy to take advantage of today's antibiotics, which can wipe out *Helicobacter pylori*, the bacterium that causes most ulcers. (Gone are the days when stress, all by itself, was thought to wear holes in the stomach.) If *H. pylori* is the culprit in your case, you'll probably get a 10- to 14-day course of treatment. Complete recovery takes about eight weeks. In the meantime, there are many steps you can take to relieve discomfort and prevent a recurrence. Don't use any of the herbal medicines until you've finished all the antibiotics.

What's wrong

Peptic ulcers are pitlike sores in the lining of your stomach or the uppermost section of your small intestine, the duodenum. They occur when pepsin, a digestive enzyme, begins to digest your own tissue. Your gastrointestinal (GI) tract usually protects itself from digestive juices with a thick layer of mucus and natural antacids. But bacteria that might be living in the wall of your GI tract, called *Helicobacter pylori,* can break down this defense system. So can long-term use of nonsteroidal anti-inflammatory drugs such as aspirin and ibuprofen.

Put Acid in Neutral

⌁ The quickest and easiest pain relievers are over-the-counter **antacids**, such as Maalox or Mylanta, which will help neutralize stomach acid, and **H₂ blockers**, such as Tagamet, Pepcid, Axid, and Zantac, which reduce stomach acid secretion. In fact, these drugs may even heal your ulcer over time. For antacids, take two tablespoons after every meal, at bedtime, and any other time you feel your ulcer starting to act up. With H_2 blockers, follow label directions. If you begin to get constipated or show signs of diarrhea, you're overmedicating. Try cutting the dose in half.

⌁ **Eating** may also help temporarily relieve your discomfort. That's because your stomach acid becomes neutralized as food is digested. But if you have a duodenal ulcer, eating will actually make your pain worse . . . *unless* you eat a high-fiber diet. Fiber slows down the digestive process. Duodenal pain is alleviated when food travels more slowly through the stomach, allowing more time for stomach acid to be neutralized.

⌁ Some animal studies suggest that **ginger** may help reduce the release of digestive fluids in the GI tract. It also works against inflammation. You can swallow capsules or break them open and dissolve them in water or juice. Take no more than 1 teaspoon per day, as too much can have a reverse effect and cause irritation. You can try eating some candied ginger (available in health-food stores). Commercial ginger ales probably don't contain enough ginger to do much good.

Don a Protective Coat

🔺 Licorice, which forms a protective coating between your stomach lining and your stomach acid, has been proven to help ulcers heal. Make sure you use a form of licorice known as **deglycyrrhizinated licorice (DGL)**, since regular licorice can send your blood pressure through the roof. Chew one or two DGL wafers about 30 minutes before each meal. You shouldn't take it if you're still on antibiotics. (*Off-limits* . . . if you use any kind of snuff or chewing tobacco containing licorice filler. You might put too much licorice in your system.)

🔺 Also used to coat sore throats, the inner bark of the **slippery elm** produces a lot of mucilage, a transparent, sticky, gelatinous substance, which can help protect the lining of your stomach. As long as you're not taking medication, you can take 700 milligrams of slippery elm in capsule form after every meal. Or, if you prefer to take it in tea form, steep 1 to 2 teaspoons of the dried bark in a cup of hot water for 20 to 30 minutes, then strain. Drink three cups a day.

🔺 Chew and swallow a teaspoon of **flaxseed**. Like slippery elm, the seeds create a soothing mucilage in the stomach. And they're a top-notch source of heart-healthy omega-3 fatty acids, which will help lower your cholesterol.

🔺 Try **aloe vera juice**. A popular European folk remedy for ulcers, the juice seems to quell gastrointestinal inflammation and may reduce stomach acid secretions. Drink one-third cup three times a day.

Favor Ulcer-Fighting Foods

🔺 Indulge in some **raw-cabbage juice**. It's probably not your beverage of choice, but if you have a peptic ulcer, it might hit the spot. Folk healers used it for years before a 1950s research team at Stanford University, led by Dr. Garnett Cheney, M.D., showed it to be an effective treatment. In one of the follow-up studies that confirmed Cheney's findings, people's ulcers disappeared in only seven days. The active substance in cabbage is probably glutamine, an amino acid that nourishes cells of the GI tract. If you don't have a home juicer,

Should I call
the doctor?

See a doctor if you have any ulcer symptoms—a burning sensation in your belly, belching, bloating, pain, red blood in your stool, black blood in your stool (indicating digested blood), or unexplained nausea. If you vomit blood (which looks like dark or black coffee grounds, or is bright red or maroon), have tarry black stool (which indicates internal bleeding), or feel extreme pain, your ulcer may have perforated—that is, opened a hole all the way through the stomach or duodenum. This development could be life threatening. See a doctor or get to the emergency room immediately.

Skip it!

People say it works. Seems like it should work. Even kind of feels like it works. What is it? Plain old milk. Once thought to soothe ulcer pain, milk actually increases production of stomach acid, so in the long run, it will make you feel worse rather than better.

you can pick up raw-cabbage juice in health-food stores. Drink a quart every day for three weeks for best results.

↝ Do you hate cabbage? **Pineapple** is another good source of glutamine.

↝ Eat plenty of **onions**. They contain sulfur compounds that may help to neutralize *H. pylori*.

↝ Help yourself to **honey**. Some studies show that honey can discourage the growth of ulcer-causing *H. pylori* bacteria. Spread some honey on your morning toast, use it instead of sugar on cereal, or add it as sweetener to herbal teas.

Honor Other Herbals

↝ **Astragalus** is an immune enhancer, natural antibiotic, and anti-inflammatory that you can use when you're not taking antibiotics. Take 2 grams in capsule form every day.

↝ Another member of the ginger family, **turmeric**, also seems to protect the gastrointestinal lining, and it also reduces gas. Take one-third teaspoon of powdered root between meals, or use it to season your food. (Turmeric doesn't make a good tea because it won't dissolve in water.) Don't overdo it, as too much turmeric can upset your digestive system rather than help it. (*Off-limits* . . . if you have gallstones. Excessive turmeric can make them worse.)

Put the Kettle On

↝ **Chamomile tea** is an old-time favorite for soothing the stomach because it calms inflammation. Pour a half-cup boiling water over 2 teaspoons chopped flowers. Steep for 5 minutes, then strain.

↝ **Peppermint** is another anti-inflammatory that can relieve pain and help you heal. To make tea, pour one cup of boiling water over a tablespoon of chopped leaves, steep for a couple of minutes, then strain out the leaves. (*Off-limits* . . . if you have a problem with gastroesophageal reflux disease, which can be aggravated by peppermint.)

Cease Stressing

↝ Practice **deep breathing**, **meditate**, listen to soothing **music**, practice **yoga**, inhale **calming scents**—whatever you can do to take the edge off the stress in your life. In the days before we knew about *H. pylori*, ulcers were thought to result from excessive emotional stress. Now we know better, but doctors have found that stress can trigger pain by increasing production of stomach acid. And if you already have *H. pylori* in your system, the opportunistic bacteria take advantage of your reduced defenses—and get started on ulcer formation.

If you're going through a particularly tough period, spring for a weekly **massage**. There's no more enjoyable way to relax and melt away stress.

The Power of Prevention

Vitamin C may slow down the growth of *H. pylori* if you have colonies of these bacteria in your stomach. Take a 1,000-milligram supplement twice a day. Citrus fruits and vegetables, especially tomatoes, are good dietary sources.

Vitamin A is a must. People who get plenty of it are the least likely to develop duodenal ulcers. Try to get at least 10,000 IU a day, in a combination of supplements and diet. The best way to consume enough vitamin A is to add a broad range of fruits and vegetables to your diet and take a daily multivitamin.

Eat plenty of **yogurt** containing active cultures, especially *Lactobacillus acidophilus,* beneficial bacteria that inhibit *H. pylori*. It's an especially good idea to eat plenty of yogurt while you're taking antibiotics, since these drugs diminish the levels of the "good" bacteria in your gut that keep "bad" bacteria in check.

Go easy on alcohol, which can irritate the stomach lining. Two 3-ounce glasses of wine a day for a man and one for a woman are the limits.

Be moderate in your use of **aspirin, ibuprofen**, and other nonsteroidal anti-inflammatory drugs. They can contribute to ulcer formation.

Avoid caffeine and tobacco. Both increase production of stomach acid, and tobacco makes antibiotics less effective.

Old **wives' tale**

Doctors used to think spicy foods were a no-no for people who have peptic ulcers. Modern research, however, has shown that this isn't necessarily so. In fact, there's some evidence to suggest that hot peppers, which contain a chemical called capsaicin, may actually help to heal ulcers by stimulating blood flow to the wound.

Urinary Tract Infections

You know that burning sensation when you urinate means another urinary tract infection. One in five women suffer from at least one such infection at least once a year. If your doctor has prescribed antibiotics, it's important to finish all the pills. But in the meantime, drink your cranberry juice—it really does work—and follow these other steps to cut short an infection and ease its sting.

What's wrong

Women get urinary tract infections (UTIs)—a term that includes bladder infections—much more often than men. Often the problem is a combination of cystitis, an infection of the bladder, and urethritis, an infection of the urethra. UTIs typically occur after bacteria in the anal area get pushed into the urethra, often during intercourse. UTIs are more likely to occur after menopause, since tissues in the vagina and urethra grow thinner and drier and are more prone to infection. Symptoms include fever, burning during urination, a feeling of bladder fullness, and frequent need to urinate. Men usually get UTIs as a consequence of a swollen prostate gland, which obstructs their urine flow.

Drink Up

At the first sign of infection, mix a cold and frothy drink with **baking soda**. Dissolve one-quarter teaspoon of baking soda in 4 ounces of water. Drink two glasses of water, then the mixed drink. The baking soda helps create a more alkaline (less acidic) environment in your bladder, making it more difficult for bacteria to thrive.

Throughout the day, have a **glass of water every hour** or so. When you flood your urinary tract with water, you flush out bacteria. Also, the more water you drink, the more you dilute your urine, so it's less irritating.

It's not an old wives' tale: Research has shown that **cranberry juice** does help women get rid of urinary tract infections faster. (It also helps prevent them.) There's nothing in the juice to stop bacteria from multiplying, but it does contain an acid that prevents bacteria from sticking to the lining of the urinary tract. If they don't stick, they are easily flushed away by your urine. Drink an 8-ounce glass daily, both as a way to prevent UTIs and to treat them.

Avoid citrus drinks, tomato juice, coffee, and **alcohol.** All of these drinks may make urination more painful.

Steep Well

Help yourself to **garlic tea**. Garlic contains powerful bacteria-killing compounds that make it ideal for battling the bugs that cause UTIs. Peel a couple of fresh garlic cloves, mash them well, then drop them in warm water. Let them steep for five minutes. Alternatively, you can make a tea by stirring a teaspoon of garlic powder in hot water.

To help your immune system fight the infection—and boost your fluid intake at the same time—make **echinacea tea** using tea bags or by steeping 2 teaspoons of the raw root in hot water. Drink three cups of tea a day.

Make a tea of **lovage** (a member of the carrot family) by pouring a cup of boiling water over 2 teaspoons of minced, dried root. Steep for 10 minutes, then strain and drink. This garden herb contains components with anti-inflammatory and bacteria-killing powers.

Try drinking **nettle tea**. Nettle is a diuretic. It will make you urinate more, which will help flush bacteria out of your system. Use 1 teaspoon of the dried herb and steep in a cup of hot water. Drink one cup a day.

Herbal Antiseptics

Uva ursi (also called bearberry because bears like its red berries) is a short shrub whose leaves have been used for hundreds of years to treat urinary tract infections because of their antiseptic properties. If you take capsules containing powdered leaves, you'll need 500 to 1,000 milligrams three times a day. If you use a standardized extract, take 125 to 250 milligrams three times a day. Stop taking this herb when you feel well again, since it may not be safe for long-term use. If you're taking uva ursi, don't also take vitamin C; it will make your urine more acidic, which will compromise the effects of the herb.

Goldenseal is a natural weapon against the *E. coli* bacteria, the culprit behind so many cases of UTIs. It not only fights the bacteria, but also stimulates your immune system and helps heal inflammation in the urinary tract. Take 500 to 1,000 milligrams of goldenseal-root extract once a day for up to a week.

The Power of Prevention

Vitamin C, vitamin A, and **bioflavonoids** all render your bladder more impervious to clinging bacteria. Take 1,000 to 1,400 milligrams of vitamin C and 300 to 600 milligrams of bioflavonoids daily. A helpful dose of vitamin A is 50,000 IU daily, but this much can be toxic over long periods and requires a doctor's supervision.

Did you **know?**

Even though few men suffer from urinary tract infections, any male with an enlarged prostate has a higher-than-average risk. Fortunately, there are a number of remedies that can help manage this problem. (See Prostate Enlargement, page 198).

🔖 If you use spermicides or a diaphragm, consider **another type of birth control**. These can contribute to UTIs by altering the bacteria in the vagina, which can then get into the urethra.

🔖 Many doctors advise women to **wash their genitals** before sex and **urinate afterward**. Urine will flush away bacteria that can be pushed up into the urethra during intercourse.

🔖 When underwear is warm and damp, it's an ideal breeding place for bacteria. Instead of synthetics, wear loose-fitting **cotton underwear** that "breathes."

🔖 For the same reason, don't loiter in a wet, tight-fitting bathing suit. Change into **dry clothes** as soon as possible after you take a swim.

🔖 A recent Finnish study found that women who frequently eat **cheese and yogurt** have fewer UTIs, possibly because these foods contain beneficial bacteria that help keep troublesome bacteria in check.

Warts

You don't have to touch a toad to get a wart—and you don't have to see a doctor to get rid of one, although there are several medical approaches to doing so. Warts can be frozen with a squirt of liquid nitrogen or burned off using lasers or an electric needle. At the pharmacy, you'll find several wart cures, including liquids and plasters containing salicylic acid, which has a peeling effect. (They can be harsh, so be sure to follow the directions on the label.) In the panoply of wart-removal techniques, however, these are only the tip of the iceberg. In fact, folk remedies for warts could fill an entire book. Here are some of the best.

Irritate Warts to Death

➤ Cover the wart with a small piece of **duct tape**. According to a recent study, duct tape works even better against warts than cryotherapy (using liquid nitrogen to freeze them off). Cut a piece that will just cover the wart. Stick it on and leave it there for six days. When you take the tape off, soak the area in water for a few minutes, then use a disposable emery board or pumice stone to file down the dead, thick skin. Leave the wart uncovered overnight and apply a new patch in the morning. Repeat the procedure until you're wart-free. How does duct tape help? It's likely that the mild skin irritation it causes spurs your immune system to fight off the virus once and for all.

➤ Apply freshly crushed **garlic** directly to the wart and cover with a bandage. The caustic effect of the garlic will cause the wart to blister and fall off in as little as one week. Apply new garlic every day, avoiding contact with healthy surrounding skin. (Smearing the area around the wart with **petroleum jelly** can help.) For an added effect, some herbalists suggest eating raw garlic or taking three garlic capsules a day to help the immune system fight the virus.

➤ Apply a compress or cotton ball soaked in **vinegar** and tape it down on the wart with an elastic bandage for at least one or two hours daily.

➤ Pull a **dandelion** from your yard, break the stem, and

What's **wrong**

If you have a wart, it means the human papillomavirus (HPV) has invaded a tiny cut in the skin. HPV is really an umbrella term for many strains of a virus that can show up all over the body. Some types of warts are found singly; others, in clusters. Generally, the wart appears as a pale skin growth with a rough surface. Plantar warts, which grow on the bottom of the feet, can be so painful that walking is difficult. Genital warts, found around the genital and anal area, are very contagious and can increase the risk of cervical, penile, and other cancers.

Should I call
the doctor?

Genital warts require immediate medical attention, and if your partner has them, you both need treatment. They are potentially serious and should never be treated exclusively with home remedies or OTCs. But the warts that appear on other parts of your body are not dangerous, and you can try any number of remedies before turning to a doctor or dermatologist. If you're over 45 and develop a new wart, however, it's a good idea to get the growth looked at by a doctor to rule out skin cancer.

squeeze some of its liquid onto your wart. Do this daily as needed. The sap is mildly irritating, so it stimulates your immune system to take care of the wart. Don't use dandelions that have been treated with herbicides during the previous few years.

Acidic Approaches

⬧ Grind up a few **vitamin C** tablets, mix with enough water to make a paste, and dab it onto your wart. Cover the paste with a bandage or tape. Because the tablets are highly acidic, they can help wear the wart away and also fight the virus itself.

⬧ If a piece of **birch bark** is available, dampen it with water, and tape it over your wart with the inner side of the bark facing your skin. The bark contains salicylates, which are also found in many over-the-counter wart treatments.

⬧ You can also make a tea from **powdered birch bark**, available from health-food stores. Steep a teaspoon of bark in a cup of boiling water for 10 minutes, let it cool, soak a cloth in it, and press it on the wart.

Kitchen Cures

⬧ Tape a piece of **banana peel**, inner side down, over the wart before you go to bed. A chemical in the peel can slowly dissolve the wart.

⬧ Do the same with a piece of **lemon peel**. An oil in the peel seems to discourage warts.

⬧ **Papaya** contains an enzyme that digests dead tissue. Make shallow cuts on the surface of an unripe papaya, collect the sap that runs out, and let it coagulate. Mix the thickened sap with water, then apply morning and night.

⬧ A popular folk remedy is to rub a juicy, freshly cut slice of **raw potato** over a wart. (Pennsylvania Dutch tradition says this remedy won't work unless you bury the used potato, but others report no need to give the spud a send-off.) We can't vouch for the efficacy of this cure, but it can't hurt.

⬧ Crush a fresh **basil** leaf and tape it over your wart with waterproof first-aid tape (or even regular tape in a pinch). The leaves contain virus-killing compounds. Replace with fresh basil daily for up to a week.

Imagining Warts Away

The power of suggestion has proved to be amazingly useful in making warts disappear. Odd folk remedies over the years have included rubbing the wart with dung, saliva, a penny, or raw meat—and many actually seem to work!

One doctor pretended to bombard a patient's warts with powerful X rays. Although the man was in fact given no radiation at all, his warts fell off the next day. Spend a few minutes each day just imagining that the warts are shrinking. If your child has a wart, make up an elaborate wart-curing ritual, such as rubbing the wart with a rock, placing the rock in a box, then burying it. If your child believes it will get rid of the wart, it just might.

Rub-On Remedies

Several times a day, apply a tincture of **goldenseal**, an herb that contains compounds that fight off bacteria and viruses.

Rub **castor oil** into your wart daily. The oil can make warts disappear, perhaps by keeping them moist so the skin cells in the wart just come apart.

Vitamin E oil is also said to work against warts. Once a day, pierce a vitamin E capsule and rub the contents into the wart.

If you have an **aloe vera** plant on the windowsill, break off a leaf and squeeze a few drops of gel onto the wart. Repeat daily. Some people report success with this remedy, perhaps because of the malic acid in aloe vera gel.

Give Feet the Water Cure

Plantar warts are sensitive to heat and may disappear in a few weeks if you soak your feet in **hot** (110- to 113-degree) **water** for about 15 minutes a day, a remedy published by a medical journal in the 1960s, but long since forgotten. For an added kick, pour one part **vinegar** into four parts hot water.

The Power of Prevention

Wear sandals around swimming pools and in the locker room. Wart viruses thrive in warm, moist environments.

Be sure to **dry off your wart** after you wash your hands, to reduce the chance of the virus spreading to someone else. When warts are wet, they seem to be more contagious.

Don't scratch or pick at warts. You can transfer the virus when you scratch other areas of skin.

Wrinkles

Dermatologists have many tools for tackling those little lines that mark the passage of time. One is Retin-A, a prescription cream that increases your body's production of collagen near the surface of your skin. Chemical peels use acid to burn away the top layers of wrinkled skin. And injections of the toxin Botox paralyze facial muscles temporarily so you can't wrinkle your skin with certain facial expressions. But perhaps the best option is to protect your skin just as it is, and help keep it healthy.

What's wrong

After the age of 30 or so, some of the connective tissue in your skin starts to break down, oil production slows down, and wrinkles develop. Those are facts of life. But wrinkles are also caused by factors that you can control. Smoking is a major culprit; it slows circulation, so your skin doesn't get as much oxygen. Sun exposure is another. The sun's ultraviolet rays do direct damage to connective fibers in the skin. And they release rogue oxygen molecules called free radicals, which wreak havoc on cell membranes.

De-Etch with Acids

 Use a lotion or cream that contains **alpha-hydroxy acids**, or AHAs. AHAs come from milk, fruit, and sugarcane, and clear away dead cells on the surface of your skin. These products encourage collagen growth, which fills in wrinkles. They also counteract free radicals, which are rogue oxygen molecules in your body that can damage your skin. Since AHAs can sometimes cause irritation, try a touch of the product on a small patch of skin first. If the patch doesn't turn red by the next day, the moisturizer is safe for you to use.

 Soak a washcloth in **milk** and apply it to your skin. Milk contains alpha-hydroxy acids.

 Apply fresh **aloe vera gel**, which contains malic acid. Cut off a leaf at the base and slit it open with a knife. Scrape out the gel with a spoon, taking care not to rupture the green rind, and apply.

 Papayas are chock-full of enzymes that can etch away the top layer of your skin, reducing the appearance of wrinkles. Wash and peel a papaya, then thoroughly mix two tablespoons of it with a tablespoon of dry oatmeal to help exfoliate your skin. Apply it to your skin and leave it on for 10 minutes. Scrub off the mixture with a washcloth.

Plump Up Skin

 Apply a **moisturizer** every morning. When you add moisturizer, dry skin expands a bit, which helps hide the wrinkles. Also, moisturizers make your skin softer and more elastic.

🍃 Try an **avocado** facial for moisture as well as **vitamin E**, an antioxidant. Puree the pulp, smooth it on your face, and leave it on for 20 minutes.

Eat , Sleep, and Move for Smoother Skin

🍃 Eat fish like **salmon, sardines, tuna**, and **mackerel** several times a week. These are rich in omega-3 fatty acids, which are very nourishing to your skin.

🍃 Another good way to get omega-3s into your diet is to eat a teaspoon of **flaxseed oil** each day. You can mix the oil with juice or cereal, or drizzle it over a salad.

🍃 Pile your plate with plenty of **fruits, vegetables, nuts**, and **seeds**. These offer vitamins A, C, and E—antioxidants that block harmful free radicals before they can cause skin damage.

🍃 Even if you're getting more **vitamin C** in your diet, go a step further by putting it directly on skin. Research presented at a recent international dermatology conference shows that using 5% vitamin C cream can boost the skin's production of collagen and help erase signs of aging after six months.

🍃 Get in the habit of **sleeping on your back**. When you sleep on your side or stomach, you bury your face into the pillow, "pressing in" wrinkles and crevices.

🍃 **Exercise** 20 to 30 minutes most days of the week. Maybe you've noticed that exercise can cause flushing—a sure sign that oxygen and nourishment in your blood are reaching the capillaries in your skin.

The Power of Prevention

🍃 **Don't smoke**.

🍃 Drink enough **water** so that your urine is very pale. Drinking a lot of water really does help keep your skin moist.

🍃 Every day, apply **sunscreen** to your face, neck, and other areas of exposed skin before you head outdoors.

🍃 **Never use a tanning salon**. A half-hour there does more damage than lying on the beach all day without sunscreen.

🍃 Wear **sunglasses** to avoid wrinkles around your eyes, aka crow's-feet. The wrinkles come from squinting. Even if you've already started to have crow's-feet, the lines can disappear after several months of consistently wearing sunglasses.

Should I call
the doctor?

If you'd like to see more improvements than you're getting from self-help treatments, talk to your doctor or a dermatologist about medical options for treating your wrinkles.

Skip it!

Will goofy facial exercises treat wrinkles? Some beauty books and magazines claim so. But smiles, grimaces, and other facial contortions just contribute to further wrinkling.

Yeast Infections

Most women suffer the itching and discomfort of a vaginal yeast infection at least once in their lives. Some of them get them often enough that they know the symptoms at once and head to the drugstore for an over-the-counter antifungal cream such as Gyne-Lotrimin or Monistat. (If you need a stronger treatment, your doctor can prescribe an oral antifungal drug.) Whatever medication you're taking, other measures are also helpful, not only for treating vaginal infections but also for preventing a recurrence. Most of the remedies in this chapter are specifically for *vaginal* infections.

What's wrong

We all carry small amounts of yeast. Called *Candida albicans*, it inhabits various moist parts of our bodies, usually without causing problems. But occasionally something triggers yeast cells to multiply. One trigger is antibiotics, which can kill off beneficial bacteria that keep yeast populations in check. Most women will have a vaginal yeast infection at some point in their lives. Symptoms include itching, redness, and a white, lumpy discharge (sometimes with an unpleasant smell). Another type of yeast infection, thrush, occurs in the throat, and can afflict both men and women.

Rinse or Soak

Douche twice a day, for two days in a row, with a mixture of 2 tablespoons white **vinegar** in 1 quart water. This slightly acidic solution creates an environment that's unwelcome to yeast. But you should only do this for two days, and only when you have a yeast infection. If you use a vinegar douche when you don't need to, you actually rinse out the beneficial bacteria that keep infections at bay.

Sprinkle a cup of **sea salt** in a tub of warm water, stir the water around until the salt dissolves, then take a nice soak. You can do this every day, as long as it helps relieve itching and pain. The saltwater soak also speeds up healing.

Pick the Stinking Rose

Eat a few cloves of **garlic** each day. "The stinking rose," as it's sometimes called, has been used for several millennia to combat everything from colds to intestinal infections. Its antifungal action makes it useful against yeast infections. It's most effective if crushed and eaten raw. If you don't relish the idea of eating a whole clove, chop it up and sprinkle it on salads, or stir it into pasta sauce.

Some people recommend inserting a gauze-wrapped garlic clove into the vagina. But most women will prefer using an **antifungal cream**—especially since the garlic can sting.

Battle Yeast with Bacteria

🌿 Every day, eat a cup of plain, unsweetened **yogurt** that contains live *Lactobacillus acidophilus* bacteria. *L. acidophilus* has been shown to cut down on yeast overgrowth in the vagina and the intestines. Note that if what you have is a bacterial infection and not a yeast infection, yogurt will actually make matters worse.

🌿 Buy capsules or tablets of *Lactobacillus acidophilus*. Look for a supplement that contains one billion to two billion live organisms per pill. You can either take two pills daily, or you can use the supplement as a vaginal suppository. (To help prevent infection, many women use a single dose of acidophilus every month on the last day of their menstrual period.)

Other Fungus Fighters

🌿 Prepare a solution of **cinnamon**, which research suggests has strong antifungal properties. (In fact, German researchers concluded that impregnating toilet paper with cinnamon would completely suppress the fungus responsible for yeast infections.) Add 8 to 10 broken sticks of cinnamon to 4 cups of boiling water and let them simmer for about 5 minutes. Take the pot off the burner and let the cinnamon steep for about 45 minutes. Some herbalists suggest using the lukewarm solution as a douche, but others say drinking cinnamon tea can also help control yeast infections.

🌿 Try supplements of **lapacho tree bark** (also known as **pau d'arco** and **taheebo**), which is thought to be a potent infection fighter. (It's even been researched as an anti-cancer agent.) You can make a tea by boiling 2 tablespoons of the herb in 1 quart of water and storing it in the refrigerator before straining and drinking. But some natural medicine practitioners say certain ingredients in the bark don't dissolve in water, making capsules more effective. A standard dose is 300 milligrams taken three times daily.

🌿 To help your immune system fight the infection, take three 200-milligram doses of **echinacea** three times a day, or a dropper of tincture in a half-cup of water four times a day. Take echinacea daily for up to two weeks, then stop taking it for two weeks.

Should I call **the doctor?**

If you're a woman who has been previously treated for vaginal yeast infections, you're probably familiar with the symptoms, and can treat them on your own. Otherwise, always see a doctor to rule out other problems, such as a sexually transmitted disease. You should also get medical care if you have a discharge that's bloody or very foul-smelling, feel pain during urination or intercourse, or have symptoms that don't go away after you've been treating them for five days. And if you've been taking antibiotics for another infection, talk to your doctor about an alternative treatment, since use of antibiotics is often associated with yeast infections.

To Eat and Not to Eat

When you have an infection, cut way back on sugary foods and starches. **Avoid white bread, pasta, honey, molasses, and fruit juices**. These foods raise the level of blood sugar (glucose) in your body, and yeast feeds on glucose.

Avoid alcohol. Yeast digests alcohol too—and you don't want well-fed yeast if you're trying to end an infection.

The Power of Prevention

Go without underwear at night. Since yeast flourishes in warm, moist environments, the ventilation will help you avoid infections. When you do wear underwear, go with cotton or with cotton-lined panties. They allow for better air circulation than synthetic fibers.

For the same reason, **leave tight pants in the closet**.

Don't linger in a wet bathing suit after swimming. Shower promptly and change into dry clothes.

Use a **hair dryer** on cool setting (never hot!) to dry the external vaginal area completely after you've been bathing or swimming.

Don't use soap or very hot water to cleanse the vaginal tissues. If you do, you'll remove healthy natural skin barriers that help to control yeast.

Refrain from using scented tampons, feminine deodorants, and douches. The chemical used to create pleasant fragrances can upset the delicate environment in the vagina and allow yeast to take over.

Also **avoid perfumed dusting powders**. Some women develop an irritation when using these powders—and the additional irritation makes them more prone to yeast infection.

Make a point of **urinating after intercourse**. Mucous membranes of the vagina normally are slightly acidic, but semen is alkaline, making it friendlier to yeast. Urinating will help make the area less inviting to infectious growth.

Cautions and Side Effects

Supplements are helpful for scores of health problems, but just as with drugs, you need to use care when taking them. Yes, even herbs and other harmless-seeming substances can have unwanted side effects if you use them inappropriately. Before you take an herb or a supplement recommended in this book, check the information below to learn about cautions to keep in mind. If you experience any side effects while taking a supplement, stop taking it and contact your doctor right away.

ACIDOPHILUS At first, may increase gassiness or bloating. Amounts exceeding 10 billion viable organisms daily may cause mild intestinal problems. If taking antibiotics, wait at least two hours before taking an acidophilus supplement.

ANISE Do not take anise during pregnancy.

ARGININE Take only under the guidance of a knowledgeable medical doctor. High doses may cause nausea and diarrhea. Do not take if you have genital herpes; may increase herpes outbreaks. Long-term effects are unknown. Do not take arginine and lysine at the same time. Take amino acid supplements at least 1½ hours before or after meals.

ARNICA Do not apply to broken or bleeding skin. Not to be used during pregnancy. Can cause an allergic rash in sensitive people or with prolonged use.

ASTRAGALUS Not recommended if a health condition is causing high fever or pronounced swelling.

B COMPLEX Do not exceed the dosage recommended on the label.

BETA-CAROTENE Avoid single supplements in excess of 25 milligrams daily. Larger amounts have no benefit, and may cause harm.

Avoid if you have hypothyroidism; your body may not be able to convert beta-carotene to vitamin A.

BLACK COHOSH Not to be taken by pregnant or nursing women. If you're taking estrogen therapy, consult a doctor before taking black cohosh. Do not use for more than 6 months. Do not take if you have heart disease or you're on medication for high blood pressure. May cause occasional stomach upset, diarrhea, abdominal pain, headache, lowered heart rate, and elevated blood pressure. Large doses may cause vertigo, headache, nausea, impaired vision, vomiting, and impaired circulation.

BROMELAIN May cause nausea, vomiting, diarrhea, skin rash, and heavy menstrual bleeding. May increase the risk of bleeding in people taking aspirin or blood thinners. Do not take bromelain if you are allergic to pineapple.

CALCIUM Do not exceed 2,500 milligrams daily except under a doctor's supervision. Some natural sources of calcium, such as oyster shells, bone meal, and dolomite, may be contaminated with lead; check the label to make sure it comes from "refined" or "purified" sources. High doses may cause constipation. If you have had calcium oxalate kidney stones, check with your doctor before taking calcium.

CARNITINE Take the "L" form only (L-carnitine), and only with consent of a health-care professional. The "D" form may displace the active form of carnitine in tissues and lead to muscle weakness. Doses above 2 grams may cause mild diarrhea. Use of individual amino acids in large doses is considered experimental, and long-term effects on health are unknown.

CASCARA Don't take if you're pregnant or in a weakened condition. Do not take for more than 8 days, except with a doctor's guidance. Do not use if you have intestinal inflammation, intestinal obstruction, or abdominal pain, as it may cause laxative dependency and diarrhea.

CASTOR OIL Do not use internally if you have intestinal obstruction or abdominal pain. Do not use for more than 8 days. Not to be used during pregnancy.

CATNIP Not to be used during pregnancy.

CAT'S CLAW Do not use if you have hemophilia or are pregnant. Side effects may include headache, stomachache, or difficulty breathing. This herb also has contraceptive properties.

CELERY SEED Not to be used during pregnancy. Use with caution if you have a kidney disorder. Avoid overexposure to direct sunlight when using this herb: It may make your skin more sensitive.

CHAMOMILE Taken internally, this herb can cause severe allergic reactions. Drink the tea with caution, especially if you are allergic to closely related plants, such as aster and chrysanthemum. Chamomile contains coumarin, an anticoagulant. Use with caution if you have blood-clotting disorders or take anticoagulant medications.

CHASTEBERRY May counteract the effectiveness of birth-control pills. May contain licorice or Siberian ginseng, which can elevate blood pressure. Read product labels carefully if you have high blood pressure.

CINNAMON Do not take large amounts during pregnancy.

COENZYME Q$_{10}$ Get medical advice if you take this supplement for more than 20 days at daily doses exceeding 120 milligrams. Rare side effects may include heartburn, nausea, and stomachache. (These can be prevented by taking the supplement with a meal.) May decrease the effectiveness of the blood-thinning medication warfarin (Coumadin).

COPPER Do not exceed 2 milligrams daily on a regular basis. The recommended form is copper sulfate, since copper oxide (cupric oxide) is not absorbed by the body.

CURCUMIN May cause heartburn in some people.

DANDELION Use with caution if you have gastric acidity, digestive ulcers, gallstones, blockage of the bile ducts, acute gallbladder inflammation, or intestinal blockage. If you have gallbladder disease, do not use root preparations. Do not use as a diet aid.

DEGLYCYRRHIZINATED LICORICE (DGL) Not to be used during pregnancy. If you have high blood pressure, be sure to take only the DGL form of licorice, never straight licorice. Use caution if you have high blood pressure; heart rhythm abnormalities; cardiovascular, liver, or kidney disorders; or low potassium levels. Do not use DGL more than three times a week for more than 4 to 6 weeks. Overuse may lead to water retention, high blood pressure due to potassium loss, or impaired heart and kidney function. Do not take with blood pressure, diuretic, corticosteroid, antiarrhythmic, or antihistamine medications.

DIGESTIVE ENZYMES Alpha-galactosidase supplements alter the way you process sugar: Don't use without a doctor's consent if you have diabetes. Do not use if you have galactosemia, a rare condition that causes an adverse reaction to all foods containing the sugar galactose. Do not take if you are sensitive to mold or penicillin. (Digestive enzyme supplements are often made from a type of mold.)

ECHINACEA Should not be taken if you have a chronic immune or autoimmune disease such as tuberculosis, lupus, multiple sclerosis, or rheumatoid arthritis. Avoid using in conjunction with drugs that are toxic to the liver, such as anabolic steroids, amiodarone, methotrexate, and ketoconazole, as it may worsen liver damage. Do not take echinacea if you are allergic to closely related plants, such as ragweed, asters, chrysanthemums, chamomile, and marigold. Do not use for more than 8 weeks.

ELDER, ELDERBERRY Seeds, bark, leaves, and unripe fruit may cause vomiting or severe diarrhea.

FALSE UNICORN Not to be used during pregnancy. Do not take if you are emaciated or experiencing acute inflammation. May cause gastrointestinal irritation.

FENNEL Do not use medicinally for more than 6 weeks.

FENUGREEK Not to be used during pregnancy.

FISH OIL Do not take more than 6,000 milligrams of fish oil a day, since too much can interfere with normal blood clotting. If you are taking blood thinners, such as Coumadin or heparin, or you take aspirin regularly, do not take fish-oil supplements unless advised by your physician. Not to be taken if you have a bleeding disorder, uncontrolled high blood pressure, or an allergy to any kind of fish. If you have diabetes, check with your doctor before taking fish oil because of its high fat content. Fish oil increases bleeding time, possibly resulting in nosebleeds and easy bruising, and may cause upset stomach. Don't take cod-liver oil; it is high in vitamins A and D, which can be toxic in high amounts.

FLAXSEED Do not use if you have bowel obstruction or thyroid problems. Always take with water. May decrease the absorption of medications. Heating or cooking flaxseed oil will destroy the omega-3 fatty acids in it and also cause the formation of harmful free radical oxidants. Best if taken with a meal that contains some fat.

FOLIC ACID Do not take doses above 1,000 micrograms a day without medical supervision. Excess folic acid can cause progressive nerve damage if you have a vitamin B$_{12}$ deficiency. Levels exceeding 400 micrograms can mask vitamin B$_{12}$ deficiencies.

GAMMA LINOLENIC ACID (GLA) Do not use supplements without the supervision of a physician if you are taking aspirin or anticoagulants (blood thinners) regularly, have a seizure disorder, or are taking epilepsy medication such as phenothiazines. Do not take borage oil (containing GLA) if you are pregnant or nursing. May cause headaches, indigestion, nausea, and softening of stools.

GINGER If you have gallstones, do not use the dried root or powder, which may increase bile secretion. Do not use if you are pregnant.

GINKGO BILOBA Rarely, gingko may cause headache, stomachache, or other allergic reactions, as well as restlessness or irritability (these side effects usually subside). Do not use with antidepressant MAO inhibitor drugs such as phenelzine sulfate (Nardil) or tranylcypromine (Parnate); aspirin or other non-steroidal anti-inflammatory medications; or blood-thinning medications such as warfarin (Coumadin). May cause rash, diarrhea, and vomiting in doses exceeding 240 milligrams of concentrated extract.

GINSENG If you have a heart condition, high blood pressure, or an anxiety disorder, consult your doctor before taking ginseng. May cause insomnia, nervousness, diarrhea, headaches, and high blood pressure. Has been reported to cause menstrual bleeding in post-menopausal women. Korean, Chinese, or American ginseng should not be used if you have acute illness, fever, or swelling. Don't take Siberian ginseng if you have high blood pressure or high fever. Do not take a ginseng product combined with another herbal stimulant, particularly ma huang (ephedra). When taking ginseng, restrict your intake of caffeinated beverages.

GLUCOSAMINE Glucosamine may cause nausea or heartburn. This can usually be alleviated by taking it with meals.

GLUTAMINE Do not take if you have end-stage liver failure or kidney failure.

GOLDENSEAL Should not be used for more than one week because it decreases the absorption of vitamin B$_{12}$, thereby leading to deficiency. Do not take if you are pregnant or have high blood pressure, hypoglycemia (low blood sugar), or weak digestion. Do not use if you have an autoimmune disease such as multiple sclerosis or lupus, or if you are allergic to plants in the daisy family such as chamomile and marigold.

GOTU KOLA Do not take if you are pregnant or nursing. Do not use with medications for diabetes or high blood pressure. Talk to your doctor if you are thinking of taking it for an extended period of time. Rarely, may cause rash or headache.

5-HYDROXYTRYPTOPHAN (5-HTP) Pregnant women should not take 5-HTP. It is experimental, and supplements are also reported to cause gastrointestinal distress, muscle pain, lethargy, and headaches. Some brands contain a contaminant called peak X, which may cause serious symptoms associated with eosinophilic myalgia syndrome (EMS). The following brands claim to perform tests confirming the absence of peak X: Natrol, Nature's Way, TriMedica, Country Life, and Solaray.

HAWTHORN If you have a cardiovascular condition, do not take regularly for more than a few weeks. Do not use if you have low blood pressure caused by heart valve problems. For long-term use, consult with a doctor, as it may cause problems at very high doses.

HOPS Do not take if prone to depression. Handle fresh or dried hops carefully, as they occasionally cause skin rashes.

HOREHOUND Not to be used during pregnancy.

HORSE CHESTNUT May interfere with the action of other drugs, especially blood-thinning medications such as warfarin (Coumadin). May irritate the gastrointestinal tract.

HORSERADISH Not to be taken if you have intestinal inflammation or kidney disorder. Not to be used by children under four years old.

LYSINE Experimental, and long-term effects are unknown. Use only under the supervision of a knowledgeable medical doctor. Do not take lysine and arginine at the same time, as they may cancel each other out.

MAGNESIUM Do not take if you have heart disease, arrhythmia, impaired kidney function, high blood pressure, or migraine headaches, or if you are taking diuretics. May cause diarrhea. Do not take doses exceeding 350 milligrams a day.

MANGANESE Do not exceed 10 milligrams daily.

MARSHMALLOW May slow the absorption of medications taken at the same time.

N-ACETYLCYSTEINE (NAC) Do not use if you have peptic ulcers or use drugs known to cause gastric lesions.

NETTLE Not to be taken during pregnancy Some people might experience mild stomach upset or a skin reaction.

PAPAYA ENZYMES May influence blood sugar levels. Do not use if you have diabetes.

PARSLEY Do not use large amounts (several cups a day) if you have kidney disease; it may increase urine flow. Not to be used during pregnancy.

PEPPERMINT May relax the muscle at the lower end of the esophagus, increasing the likelihood of heartburn. Use the herb cautiously if you are prone to acid reflux.

POTASSIUM Do not get more than 5,000 milligrams a day from food and supplements. Large doses of supplements are available only by prescription. Excessive potassium can upset the balance of other minerals in the body and cause potentially fatal heart and kidney problems.

PROBIOTICS May increase gassiness or bloating at first, which is a sign that the good bacteria are fermenting. Within a week or two, your body will adjust to the change.

PSYLLIUM Talk to your doctor before taking this fiber supplement, especially if you have difficulty swallowing or have serious intestinal disorders such as diverticulitis, ulcerative colitis, Crohn's disease, bowel obstruction, or if you are taking insulin (for diabetes) or any other medications. Psyllium should always be taken with water. May cause bloating or constipation.

PYGEUM AFRICANUM Consult your doctor if you're using this supplement to treat an enlarged prostate.

ROSEMARY May cause excessive menstrual bleeding in large amounts. Not to be taken during pregnancy.

S-ADENOSYL-L-METHIONE (SAM-E) May increase blood levels of homocysteine, a significant risk factor for cardiovascular disease.

ST. JOHN'S WORT May take several weeks to become effective. Can cause skin to be light-sensitive. Be sure to wear sunscreen and avoid spending extended time in direct sunlight. Do not use when pregnant. Avoid taking with alcohol, with over-the-counter cold medications, or with prescribed antidepressants. May cause high blood pressure when taken with ephedra compounds. Do not attempt to use this herb as a treatment for clinical depression. Serious depression requires proper medical care.

SAW PALMETTO If you have prostate problems, see your doctor for a diagnosis before using this supplement. Rare cases of stomach problems have been recorded.

SELENIUM Don't take more than 200 micrograms daily. Higher doses may cause fragile, thickened nails; stomach pain; diarrhea; nausea; a garlic odor on the breath and skin; a metallic taste in the mouth; a loss of sensation in the hands and feet; fatigue; and irritability. Doses of about 800 micrograms have been known to cause tissue damage. Works best with vitamin E.

SENNA Don't use for more than 8 to 10 days. Take 1 hour after other drugs, and always with water. Not to be taken during pregnancy. Do not use if you have abdominal pain, diarrhea, hemorrhoids, intestinal obstruction, or any inflammatory condition of the intestines. Not to be used by children younger than 12. Discontinue use if you have diarrhea or watery stools.

TAURINE May increase stomach acid. Do not take if you have diabetes.

VALERIAN Do not use with prescription medications such as diazepam (Valium) or amitriptyline (Elavil). Valerian should not be combined with alcoholic beverages. May intensify the effects of sleep-enhancing or mood-regulating medications. Discontinue valerian if you experience heart palpitations or nervousness, excitability, headaches, or insomnia.

VITAMIN A Do not exceed 10,000 IU per day. Possible side effects include weight loss, skin problems, bone pain, bleeding, vomiting, diarrhea, fatigue, dizziness, blurred vision, hair loss, joint pain, and enlargement of the liver and spleen. Do not take more than 5,000 IU if you are pregnant or trying to conceive.

VITAMIN B$_6$ Do not take more than 100 milligrams per day. Too much B$_6$ can cause (reversible) nerve damage. Possible side effects include a tingling sensation in the fingers and toes, pain, numbness, and weakness in the limbs, depression, and fatigue.

VITAMIN C Daily doses exceeding 1,000 milligrams may cause diarrhea. Pregnant women should never take more than 5,000 milligrams of vitamin C per day. If you have chronic renal failure or are on hemodialysis, consult a healthcare practitioner before supplementing with vitamin C. Always cut back to 100 milligrams daily at least

three days before a medical exam, as high amounts can interfere with some tests, particularly for blood in the stool and sugar in the urine. Large doses may also interfere with anticoagulant medications. Supplements made from a corn base may cause a reaction in people allergic to corn.

VITAMIN E The vitamin acts as a blood thinner. Consult your doctor before beginning supplementation in any amount if you're already taking aspirin or a blood-thinning medication such as warfarin (Coumadin). Use only with medical supervision if you are also taking ginkgo or fish-oil supplements; if you take aspirin regularly to help prevent heart disease; if you have high blood pressure, heart disease, or cancer; if you smoke; if you have had a stroke; or if you are at high risk for stroke. Although vitamin E is commonly sold in doses of 400 IU, one small study showed a possible increase in stroke risk in doses over 200 IU. Daily doses of more than 400 IU may cause headache, nausea, diarrhea, and fainting.

WILLOW BARK Do not use if you are allergic to aspirin or if you are taking a blood-thinning medication such as warfarin (Coumadin). May trigger asthma or allergies or cause gastrointestinal bleeding, liver dysfunction, blood-clotting disorders, kidney damage, or anaphylactic reactions. Willow bark may interact with barbiturates or sedatives such as aprobarbital or alprazolam, and it can cause stomach irritation when consumed with alcohol.

YARROW Rarely, handling flowers can cause a skin rash. Do not use during pregnancy.

ZINC Do not exceed 30 milligrams daily. Zinc may interfere with copper absorption. Possible side effects include suppression of the immune system, with increased susceptibility to infections. Daily doses of more than 30 milligrams may cause nausea and vomiting.

Index

A

Abreva, 79
Acetylcysteine. *See* N-acetylcysteine (NAC) uses
Acetyl-L-carnitine. *See* Carnitine uses
Acidophilus uses
    cautions and side effects, 245
    diarrhea prevention, 108
    flatulence relief, 127
    IBS relief, 177
    yeast infection treatment, 243
Acne, 22–23
Acupressure uses
    constipation relief, 92
    headache relief, 136
    nausea relief, 192
    sinusitis relief, 214
    toothache relief, 229
Affirmations, for anxiety, 34
Age spots, 24–25
Air filters and purifiers, 28, 29
Alcoholic beverage cautions. *See* specific ailments
Alcohol (isopropyl) uses
    blister relief, 53
    body odor elimination, 55
    poison ivy relief, 195
    swimmer's ear relief, 223
Allergies, 11, 26–29
Almonds, for high cholesterol, 151
Aloe vera uses
    acne relief, 23
    age spot treatment, 24
    athlete's foot relief, 43
    blister relief, 52
    canker sore relief, 70
    poison ivy relief, 196
    psoriasis relief, 203
    shingles relief, 210
    sunburn relief, 222
    tips for growing and using, 13
    ulcer relief, 231
    wart removal, 239
    wrinkle treatment, 240
Alpha-hydroxy acid uses
    acne relief, 22
    wrinkle treatment, 240

Angina, 30–31
Anise uses
    bad breath elimination, 50
    cautions and side effects, 245
    heartburn relief, 140
Antacids
    as diarrhea cause, 109
    as remedy, 70, 230
Antihistamine uses
    chicken pox relief, 77
    conjunctivitis relief, 89
    insect bite treatment, 169
    snoring prevention, 216
Anxiety, 32–34
Arcozon, for bronchitis, 59
Arginine uses
    cautions and side effects, 80, 245
    impotence treatment, 158
Arnica uses
    bruise treatment, 61, 62
    bursitis and tendinitis relief, 64
    carpal tunnel syndrome relief, 73
    cautions and side effects, 245
Aromatherapy, 16–17
Arthritis, 35–38
Artichoke extract, for high cholesterol, 153
Aspirin uses
    acne relief, 22
    callus and corn relief, 68
    cautions and side effects, 62, 194
    cold sore relief, 78
    insect sting treatment, 167
Asthma, 27, 39–41
Astragalus uses
    bronchitis relief, 58
    cautions and side effects, 245
    cold and flu relief, 81–82
    sinusitis relief, 214
    ulcer relief, 232
Athlete's foot, 42–44
Avocado uses
    cholesterol treatment, 151
    wrinkle treatment, 241

B

Back pain, 45–48
Bad breath, 49–51

Bag Balm, 99, 202
Baking powder, for shingles, 210
Baking soda uses
    athlete's foot relief, 42
    bad breath elimination, 51
    body odor elimination, 55
    canker sore relief, 71
    chicken pox relief, 76
    dry mouth relief, 111
    foot odor elimination, 129
    gum problem relief, 134
    heartburn relief, 141
    hive relief, 154
    indigestion relief, 162
    insect sting treatment, 168
    sunburn relief, 222
    UTI relief, 234
Banana uses
    insomnia relief, 171
    wart removal, 238
Basil, for warts, 238
Bay leaves, for dandruff, 101
Beano, 125
Bearberry, for UTIs, 235
Bee stings, 167–68
Beeswax, for pollen allergies, 29
Benzoyl peroxide uses
    acne relief, 22
    contraindications, 208
    foot odor elimination, 129
Bergamot oil, for chicken pox, 76
Beta-carotene, 245
Betadine, 53, 55
Bioflavonoid uses
    asthma relief, 40
    bruise prevention, 62
    earache relief, 113
    menstrual problems, 185
    nosebleed prevention, 194
    UTI relief, 235
Biotin, for brittle nails, 189–90
Birch bark, for warts, 238
Blackberry tea, for diarrhea, 106
Black cohosh uses
    cautions and side effects, 245
    menopause problems, 181
    menstrual problems, 186
Black pepper, for toothache, 228